Lab Manual to Accompany

Health Assessment in Nursing

SECOND EDITION

Janet Weber, RN, EdD
Professor
Department of Nursing
Southeast Missouri State University
Cape Girardeau, Missouri

Jane Kelley, RN, PhD
Professor
School of Nursing
University of Mississippi Medical Center
Jackson, Mississippi

Ann Sprengel, RN, EdD
Associate Professor
Department of Nursing
Southeast Missouri State University
Cape Girardeau, Missouri

LIPPINCOTT WILLIAMS & WILKINS
A **Wolters Kluwer** Company
Philadelphia • Baltimore • New York • London
Buenos Aires • Hong Kong • Sydney • Tokyo

Ancillary Editor: Deedie McMahon
Compositor: LWW
Printer/Binder: Victor Graphics

ISBN: 0-7817-3243-3

Any procedure or practice described in this book should be applied by the health care practitioner under appropriate supervision in accordance with professional standards of care used with regard to the unique circumstances that apply in each practice situation. Care has been taken to confirm the accuracy of information presented and to describe generally accepted practices. However, the authors, editors, and publisher cannot accept any responsibility for errors or omissions or for any consequences from application of the information in this book and make no warranty, express or implied, with respect to the contents of the book.

10   9   8   7   6   5   4

Preface

The *Lab Manual to Accompany Health Assessment in Nursing* can be used as a laboratory manual and study guide for the second edition of *Health Assessment in Nursing*. Each chapter corresponds to the textbook chapters, and each contains a **chapter pretest, interactive learner activities,** a **nursing history checklist,** a **physical assessment checklist,** a **chapter post-test, critical thinking questions, case studies,** and a **self-reflection and evaluation** tool. The lab manual can assist you with comprehending theoretical content, applying this content to acquiring history and physical assessment skills, and preparing for tests.

Prior to beginning study in each textbook chapter, take the **Chapter Pretest.** This test is designed to assess the information you may already know from a prior course. It tests basic information related to the content framework or the anatomy and physiology basic to each chapter. (Answers are located in the back of the book.) If you answer most of the questions correctly, proceed to the next section. Otherwise, review the basic framework content or anatomy and physiology found at the very beginning of the appropriate chapter. .

Next read the chapter and then participate in the **Learner Activities.** These activities are designed to assist you with learning the assessment skills covered in each chapter. These activities actively involve you as a learner to promote understanding and retention of chapter content.

Then you can interview your lab partner using the **Nursing History Checklist** tool provided to document findings. After practicing the physical examination on your lab partner, you can document your findings on the **Physical Assessment Checklist** tool provided. Both of these tools serve as a reminder of the steps involved in performing a thorough nursing history and physical examination. The completed checklists can also be handed into your nursing instructor to be evaluated for accuracy and completeness of client data.

To test your comprehension of the content provided, take the **Chapter Post-test.** Again, the test answers are provided in the back of the lab manual. To test your critical thinking abilities, answer the **Critical Thinking Questions** found after the post-test. One or two case studies follow this section to test your ability to apply new knowledge in analyzing the client data you documented from a health history interview and physical examination.

Finally, use the **Self-Reflection and Evaluation** tool to identify the degree to which you have met each of the chapter **learning objectives.** This self-evaluation will help you identify those parts of the chapter you need to review to fully comprehend the knowledge needed to effectively perform a client nursing history and physical examination.

We hope and believe this lab manual will assist you to actively learn the content and skills needed to effectively perform a Client Nursing History and Physical Examination.

Best wishes and happy learning.

Janet Weber
Jane Kelley
Ann Sprengel

Contents

UNIT I

Overview of the Health Assessment Process

The Nurse's Role in Health Assessment

CHAPTER OVERVIEW

The activities and quizzes that follow are designed to enhance learning about the initial step of the nursing process. Assessment involves the collection of data on which to make a nursing judgment. In practice, nurses collect data continually, beginning with initial comprehensive assessments and continuing with ongoing partial assessments, focused or problem-oriented assessments, and emergency assessments as well.

■ Chapter Pretest

MATCHING

Match the terms in the left column with the correct descriptions in the right column.

Term	Description
_____ 1. Assessment	A. Developing a plan of nursing care and outcome criteria
_____ 2. Diagnoses	B. Carrying out the plan of care
_____ 3. Planning	C. Sensations or symptoms that can be verified only by the client (e.g., pain)
_____ 4. Implementation	D. Problem that requires the attention or assistance of other health care professionals
_____ 5. Evaluation	E. Assessing whether outcome criteria have been met and revision the plan of care if necessary
_____ 6. Nursing diagnosis	F. Collection of subjective and objective data
_____ 7. Subjective data	G. Clinical judgment about individual, family, or community responses to actual or potential health problems and life processes
_____ 8. Objective data	H. Physiologic complications that nurses monitor to detect their onset or changes in status
_____ 9. Collaborative problem	I. Analysis of subjective and objective data to make a professional nursing judgment
_____ 10. Referral problem	J. Findings directly observed or indirectly observed through measurements (e.g., body temperature)

■ Learner Activities

WORKING WITH PEERS IN LEARNING LAB

After reading Chapter 1 in the text Health Assessment in Nursing, *2nd edition, participate in the following activities with your lab partner as assigned.*

1. Assess your lab partner's dietary intake for yesterday and also his or her satisfaction with the intake.

2. Share with your lab partner the last time you went to a physician. Describe your reason for seeing the physician. What examinations did the physician perform? What conclusions were made? Discuss how the focus of a nursing assessment would differ from the physician's assessment. Discuss how the conclusions would differ.

3. Make an observation about your lab partner. Now make a judgment based on that observation, and validate the observation with your partner. For example, "You look tired today. Describe to me your patterns of sleeping and resting."

4. Role-play how Florence Nightingale would have performed a nursing assessment in her era. Then role-play how a nurse today would approach that assessment from a different perspective (example: type of equipment used, type of questions asked). Next, brainstorm with your lab partner how a nursing assessment might change in the future—20 years from now.

■ Chapter Post-test

MULTIPLE CHOICE

Choose one best answer for each of the following multiple-choice questions.

_____ 1. A medical examination differs from a comprehensive nursing examination in that the medical examination focuses primarily on the client's

    A. physiologic status.

    B. holistic wellness status.

    C. developmental history.

    D. level of functioning.

_____ 2. The end result of a nursing assessment is the

    A. prescription of treatment.

    B. documentation of the need for a referral.

    C. client's physiologic status.

    D. formulation of nursing diagnoses.

_____ 3. Although the assessment phase of the nursing process precedes the other phases, the assessment phase is

    A. continuous.

    B. completed on admission.

    C. linear.

    D. performed only by nurses.

_____ 4. When a client first enters the hospital for an elective surgical procedure, the nurse should perform an assessment termed

    A. entry.

    B. exploratory.

    C. focused.

    D. comprehensive.

_____ 5. An ongoing or partial assessment of a client

    A. focuses on a specific problem of the client.

    B. includes a comprehensive overview of all body systems.

    C. is usually performed by another health care worker.

    D. includes a brief reassessment of the client's normal body system.

_____ 6. To prepare for the assessment of a client visiting a neighborhood
health care clinic, the nurse should first

    A. discuss the client's symptoms with other team members.

    B. plan for potential laboratory procedures.

    C. review the client's health care record.

    D. determine potential health care resources.

_____ 7. The nurse is preparing to meet a client in the clinic for the first time.
After reviewing the client's record, the nurse should

    A. analyze data that have already been collected.

    B. review any past collaborative problems.

    C. avoid premature judgments about the client.

    D. consult with the client's family members.

_____ 8. Before beginning a comprehensive health assessment of an adult client,
the nurse should explain to the client that the purpose of the assessment is to

    A. arrive at conclusions about the client's health.

    B. document any physical symptoms the client may have.

    C. contribute to the medical diagnosis.

    D. validate the data collected.

_____ 9. To arrive at a nursing diagnosis or a collaborative problem, the nurse
goes through the steps of analysis of data. After proposing possible
nursing diagnoses, the nurse should next

    A. cluster the data collected.

    B. draw inferences and identify problems.

    C. document conclusions.

    D. check for the presence of defining characteristics.

_____ 10. The depth and scope of nursing assessment has expanded significantly
over the past several decades primarily because of

    A. the growing elderly population with chronic illness.

    B. rapid advances in biomedical knowledge and technology.

    C. an increase in the number of baccalaureate programs in nursing.

    D. an increase in the number of nurse practitioners.

ESSAY QUESTIONS

1. Discuss ways in which expanding technology will change the future role of the nurse in health assessment.

2. Compare and contrast a nursing assessment with a medical assessment.

■ Self-Reflection and Evaluation of Learner Objectives

After reading Chapter 1 in the text and completing the above reviews, please identify to what degree you have met each of the following chapter learning objectives. For those objectives that you have met partially or not at all, you will want to review chapter content for that learning objective.

Objective	Very much	Somewhat	Not at all
1. Explain how assessment is applicable to every situation the nurse encounters.			
2. Differentiate between a nursing assessment and a medical assessment.			
3. Describe how assessment fits into the total nursing process.			
4. List and describe the steps of the nursing process: Subjective data collection Objective data collection Validation of data Documentation of data			
5. Describe the steps of the analysis phase of the nursing process.			
6. Explain how the nurse's role in assessment has changed over the past century. Discuss what the nurse's role might be 25 years from now.			

For additional information on this book, be sure to visit *http://connection.lww.com.*

Assessment Frameworks

CHAPTER OVERVIEW

Use the questions and exercises on these pages to review the rich history and theories of nursing in general and the nursing assessment process in particular, as presented in Chapter 2 of your textbook.

■ Chapter Pretest

MATCHING

Match the following terms in the left column with the correct description in the right column.

Term	Description
_____ 1. Nursing assessment	A. Sequences of behavior (patterns) that serve as the basis for nurses to make holistic clinical judgments (i.e., health perception/management, sleep/rest patterns)
_____ 2. Medical assessment	
_____ 3. Gordon's 11 Functional Health Patterns	
_____ 4. FANCAPES	B. Focuses on state wellness and reaction to stressors
_____ 5. Nine Patterns of Unitary Man	C. Physical fitness, nutritional awareness, stress management, environmental sensitivity, self-responsibility for health
_____ 6. Five Dimensions of Wellness	
_____ 7. Dorothea Orem's Theoretical Framework	D. Data collected to identify a nursing diagnosis or collaborative problem
_____ 8. Sister Callista Roy's Adaptation Model	E. Focus on client's self-care abilities
_____ 9. Betty Neuman's Health Systems Model	F. Data collected to identify medical diagnosis
	G. Focuses on client's ability to adapt
	H. Mnemonic device used to collect data re: fluid intake, aeration, nutrition, communication, activity, pain, elimination, and socialization
	I. Framework based on Martha Roger's theory of Unitary Human Beings by which the nurse organizes data collected (i.e., exchanging, valuing, choosing)

■ Learner Activities

1. Discuss the purpose of nursing assessment and compare it with medically focused assessment.

2. Describe how nursing assessment varies when approached from the perspective of different nursing conceptual frameworks.

3. Think about your last visit to a health care professional. What questions were asked of you that really led to your diagnosis and treatment plan? Are there questions you believe should have been asked but were not asked?

4. Obtain a copy of the health history form used at your place of employment or the clinical area where you have been assigned this semester in nursing classes. Is this form based on a nursing model or a medical model? Explain.

5. Compare and contrast Functional Health Patterns and Nine Patterns of Unitary Person.

■ Chapter Post-test

MULTIPLE CHOICE

Choose one best answer for each of the following multiple-choice questions.

_____ 1. The primary purpose of a nursing assessment is to
   A. identify real and potential nursing diagnoses and interventions.
   B. gather data that are primarily related to medical symptoms.
   C. identify patterns of functioning that conform to or deviate from norms.
   D. collect data related to psychosocial symptoms.

_____ 2. A conceptual theory or model is best defined as
   A. a set of abstract, interrelated statements.
   B. the foundation for all of nursing practice.
   C. guidelines that identify specific data collection.
   D. a framework that allows for common areas of information.

_____ 3. A conceptual model that views the client as an open system in which repeated cycles of input, process, output, and feedback constitute a dynamic, organizational pattern was developed by
   A. Sister Callista Roy.
   B. Imogene King.
   C. Marjorie Gordon.
   D. Betty Newman.

_____ 4. The goal of nursing whereby the nurse seeks to reduce ineffective responses and promote adaptational ones is associated with the conceptual model developed by
   A. Sister Callista Roy.
   B. Jean Watson.
   C. Martha Rogers.
   D. Dorothea Orem.

_____ 5. A nurse who is caring for a client interacts with the client to identify problems and establish and meet goals in order to achieve the client's maximum potential for daily living. This nurse is using a conceptual nursing model developed by

A. Jean Watson.

B. Imogene King.

C. Dorothea Orem.

D. Betty Neuman.

_____ 6. A conceptual nursing model that views the client as a unified whole, possessing integrity and characteristics more than, and different from, the sum of the parts, was developed by

A. Jean Watson.

B. Dorothea Orem.

C. Myra Levin.

D. Martha Rogers.

_____ 7. The conceptual model developed by Dorothea Orem views the client as a

A. self-care agent who performs or practices activities to maintain life, health, and well-being.

B. human being continually adapting in his or her interactions with the environment.

C. personal or interpersonal system interacting in the environment.

D. valued person to be cared for, with a fully functioning integrated self.

_____ 8. During an initial assessment, the nurse is using Gordon's functional health patterns model as a framework. To assess the client's nutritional and metabolic status, an appropriate question for the nurse to ask the client is

A. "Do you eat a healthy diet every day?"

B. "Do you have enough energy to function throughout the day?"

C. "Have you recently gained weight?"

D. "What is your typical daily food intake?"

_____ 9. One of the Nine Patterns of the Unitary Person that is similar to Gordon's functional health patterns model is the pattern related to

A. values.

B. coping.

C. moving.

D. elimination.

_____ 10. The nurse uses the mnemonic FANCAPES to quickly perform an assessment of an adult client. The nurse uses the "S" in the mnemonic to assess the client's

A. sexuality pattern.

B. self-care ability.

C. swallowing ability.

D. socialization.

■ Self-Reflection and Evaluation of Learner Objectives

After reading Chapter 2 in the text and completing the above reviews, please identify to what degree you have met each of the following chapter learning objectives. For those objectives that you have met partially or not at all, you will want to review chapter content for that learning objective.

Objective	Very much	Somewhat	Not at all
1. Differentiate between the medical model and the nursing model of assessment.			
2. Describe the purpose and focus of assessment based on the nursing theory used in your classes.			
3. Discuss various frameworks that can be used to perform a nursing assessment.			

For additional information on this book, be sure to visit *http://connection.lww.com.*

The Client in Context: Culture, Family, and Community

CHAPTER OVERVIEW

The questions and activities on these pages are designed to illustrate the importance of conducting nursing assessment in light of the clients as social beings rooted in various cultures, as members of families, and as inhabitants of various communities.

■ Chapter Pretest

MULTIPLE CHOICE

Choose one best answer for each of the following multiple-choice questions.

_____ 1. When a client in considered in context, the term *context* refers to
  A. theoretic perspective.
  B. setting, environment.
  C. family history.
  D. chart content.

_____ 2. All of the following statements about systems are true *except*:
  A. A system is an interacting whole formed of many parts.
  B. A system is more complex than the individual parts.
  C. Systems interact with one another constantly.
  D. All nursing conceptual frameworks consider the interacting systems of client and context.

TRUE/FALSE

1. T F The client's culture can affect the client's health.

2. T F The client's family can affect the client's health.

3. T F Community characteristics can affect the client's health.

4. Circle the T for each descriptor that is true of culture; circle the F for each descriptor that does not apply to culture:
  a. T F learned
  b. T F shared
  c. T F universal
  d. T F transmits meaning

   e. T F defines values

   f. T F helps to interpret information

   g. T F little variation within any one culture

   h. T F culture and race are synonymous

   i. T F cultural beliefs define health and illness

5. T F Family members and nurses often differ in their definition of family.

6. T F For health care purposes, a family is who the client says it is.

7. T F A community is defined primarily by geographic location.

8. T F Emotional health is affected by the community in which the person lives.

■ Learner Activities

1. Get together with a small group of friends or lab partners to compare beliefs and behaviors related to health and illness. Make a list to see whether there is variation within the groups. Ask each group member:

   a. What do you do to stay healthy?

   b. What do you do to feel better when you have a cold?

   c. When do you seek help from a health care professional?

   d. What home remedies do you use? vitamins/minerals? herbs? yoga? tai chi? special foods or diets? alternative or complementary therapies? What home remedies do your family members use?

   e. Do you like to be left alone or have many visitors when you are ill?

   f. What do you believe causes illness?

2. Discuss how family beliefs, habits, roles, and interactions could affect your (or another family member's) health status.

3. Discuss how genetics and environment affect biologic variation.

4. Define "culture-bound syndromes." Which clients might experience them?

5. Describe your geopolitical community's effect on the community's health.

6. Describe various communities, other than geopolitical, of which you are a part. What effect do they have on your health or illness?

7. Discuss what it means for a nurse to be culturally competent and why this is essential for nursing assessment.

■ Chapter Post-test

MULTIPLE CHOICE

Choose one best answer for each of the following multiple-choice questions.

_____ 1. Ethnocentrism is defined as:

   A. the belief that one's cultural values are superior to all others.

   B. a worldview that each of us forms based on our own culture.

   C. the basis of cultural competence.

   D. a culture-bound syndrome found in many cultural groups.

_____ 2. Choose "do" or "don't" for the following behaviors to indicate their appropriateness for cultural encounters.

Do	Don't	
		a. Be aware that some nonverbal communication may be insulting to some cultural groups (e.g., direct eye contact).
		b. Assume that a person who looks and behaves much as you do has no cultural differences.
		c. Assume that a negative or hostile communication from a client is directed at you personally as an insult.
		d. Seek feedback and constructive criticism on the transcultural interactions you have with clients.
		e. Recognize and value differences.
		f. Recognize that there is variation within all cultural and ethnic groups, often more variation within than between groups.
		g. Seek many opportunities to interact with persons of different cultures, even if it makes you uncomfortable at first.

_____ 3. Suzie is a 16-year-old daughter in the Hanes family. She is the youngest of five children. She has had a series of illnesses and does not seem to be regaining her strength. She likes school but is falling behind a bit. Her mother is very attentive to her needs but does not seem overly concerned with the continuing pattern of illness. Which of the following is most likely a Hanes family belief?

   A. Fathers are not involved with their children.

   B. Education is highly valued for sons and daughters.

   C. Emotional stress from a work environment can cause both emotional and physical illness.

   D. Community is the context in which health care professionals care for clients.

_____ 4. The best reason for the nurse to assess the client's community is:

   A. There is an interaction of culture, family, and environmental systems with the client's emotional and physical systems affecting the client's health status.

   B. Pollution from an unhealthy community can affect the client's physical health.

   C. Emotional stress from a work environment can cause both emotional and physical illness.

   D. Community is the context in which health care professionals care for clients.

MATCHING

Match the terms in the left column with the correct descriptions in the right column.

Term	Description
_____ 1. Sickle-cell disease	A. "Blocked intestine," a culture-bound syndrome thought to result from a food lump sticking to the intestinal wall
_____ 2. Empacho	
_____ 3. Low salt sweat	B. Often found in black Africans and those Caucasians acclimatized to the tropics
_____ 4. Race	C. A malaria-related condition in mosquito-infested areas of the Mediterranean
_____ 5. Ethnic group	D. A result of genetic variation across a continuum associated with distance from the equator
_____ 6. Culture-bound syndrome	E. A breeding population that mates largely with its group
_____ 7. Skin color	F. Concerned with learned behavior independent of genetics or nationality
	G. Illness that is defined by a specific cultural group and may not be interpreted as an illness by other groups

■ Self-Reflection and Evaluation of Learner Objectives

After reading Chapter 3 in the text and completing the above reviews, please identify to what degree you have met each of the following chapter learning objectives. For those objectives that you have met partially or not at all, you will want to review chapter content for that learning objective.

Objective	Very much	Somewhat	Not at all
1. Explain how culture, family, and community interact to form a context for health assessment.			
2. Define *culture* and describe its basic characteristics.			
3. Describe the mechanism at work in human cultural and biologic variation.			
4. Discuss the role of culture and biologic variation in health and illness.			
5. Discuss the role of cultural competence of the caregiver in nursing assessment.			

For additional information on this book, be sure to visit *http://connection.lww.com.*

Collecting Subjective Data

CHAPTER OVERVIEW

Let the pages of this chapter help you review information about the health history interview techniques related to obtaining subjective data during the nursing assessment. Subjective data may be sensed or reported by the client or significant other people, such as family or friends or health care personnel. Subjective data are not observable or measurable.

■ Chapter Pretest

MULTIPLE CHOICE

Choose one best answer for each of the following multiple-choice questions.

_____ 1. During an interview, the nurse collects both subjective and objective data from an adult client. Subjective data would include the client's

    A. perception of pain.

    B. height.

    C. weight.

    D. temperature.

_____ 2. During an interview with an adult client, the nurse can keep the interview from going off course by

    A. using open-ended questions.

    B. rephrasing the client's statements.

    C. inferring information.

    D. using closed-ended questions.

_____ 3. The nurse has interviewed a Hispanic client with limited English skills for the first time. The nurse observes that the client is reluctant to reveal personal information and believes in a hot-cold syndrome of disease causation. The nurse should

    A. acknowledge the client's cultural differences.

    B. request a family member to interpret for the client.

    C. use slang terms to identify certain body parts.

    D. remain in a standing position during the interview.

_____ 4. For a nurse to be therapeutic with clients when dealing with sensitive issues such as terminal illness or sexuality, the nurse should have

    A. advanced preparation in this area.

    B. experience in dealing with these types of clients.

    C. knowledge of his or her own thoughts and feelings about these issues.

    D. personal experiences with death, dying, and sexuality.

_____ 5. The nurse is interviewing a client in the clinic for the first time. The client appears to have a very limited vocabulary. The nurse should plan to

    A. use very basic lay terminology.

    B. have a family member present during the interview.

    C. use standard medical terminology.

    D. show the client pictures of different symptoms, such as "Faces Pain Chart".

_____ 6. The nurse is interviewing a client in the clinic for the first time. When the client tells the nurse that he smokes "about two packs of cigarettes a day," the nurse should

    A. look at the client with a frown.

    B. tell the client that he is spending a lot of money foolishly.

    C. provide the client with a list of dangers associated with smoking.

    D. encourage the client to quit smoking.

_____ 7. During the client interview, the nurse uses nonverbal expressions appropriately when the nurse

    A. avoids excessive eye contact with the client.

    B. remains expressionless throughout the interview.

    C. uses touch in a friendly manner to establish rapport.

    D. displays mental distancing during the interview.

_____ 8. During the interview of an adult client, the nurse should

    A. use leading questions for valid responses.

    B. provide the client with information as questions arise.

    C. read each question carefully from the history form.

    D. complete the interview as quickly as possible.

_____ 9. While interviewing a client for the first time, the nurse is using a standardized nursing history form. The nurse should

    A. maintain eye contact while asking the questions from the form.

    B. read the questions verbatim from the form.

    C. ask the client to complete the form.

    D. ask leading questions throughout the interview.

_____ 10. The nurse is interviewing a 78-year-old client for the first time. The nurse should first

    A. assess the client's hearing acuity.

    B. establish rapport with the client.

    C. obtain biographic data.

    D. use medical terminology appropriately.

■ Learner Activities

1. Obtain permission to observe client interviews in a clinic. Observe the clients' nonverbal communications. Notice the different nonverbal responses of the client. Notice differences between male and female, elderly and young, and ethnically different clients.

2. Practice using the COLDSPA mnemonic with peers or friends who are experiencing pain or other symptoms.

3. Read the section in the text on verbal communications to avoid. Give examples of each, and describe how each blocks effective communication.

4. Practice with a peer or lab partner collecting information from a selected portion of the health history. First, use the structural form and questions for the section. Next, repeat data collection for the section, but this time do not use any structured questions. Use only broad, open-ended questions, such as "Tell me about . . ." and "Can you think of anything else?"

5. Collect a complete health history, using the health history portion of the nursing assessment tool in the textbook (Appendix A: Sample Adult Nursing Health History and Physical Assessment) to obtain a complete health history on a lab partner or peer.

CASE STUDY

Read the following and analyze how the client's lifestyle might affect her health.

Stacey Kline is a 29-year-old graphic artist. She is single and lives in a one-bedroom apartment in the city. She has an extensive social network in the city and goes out to clubs and bars until at least midnight about four nights a week. Her work is very fulfilling for her, and she rates her stress level as moderate. She eats two meals a day (usually out), drinks "a lot" of coffee, smokes a pack of "light" cigarettes a day, and drinks whenever she goes out with friends. Stacey does not have a serious boyfriend at present, but she is taking birth control pills "to prevent a disaster with some guy I don't care about." She has a good supportive relationship with her family, who live 15 minutes away. She visits them at least twice a week. She is Roman Catholic and tries to go to mass every other week. She says that her faith is important to her but that it doesn't rule her life.

■ Chapter Post-test

MULTIPLE CHOICE

Choose one best answer for each of the following multiple-choice questions.

_____ 1. During an interview with an adult client for the first time, the nurse can clarify the client's statements by
   A. offering a "laundry list" of descriptors.
   B. rephrasing the client's statements.
   C. repeating verbatim what the client has said.
   D. inferring what the client's statements mean.

_____ 2. During the interview between a nurse and a client, the nurse and the client collaborate to identify problems and goals. This occurs during the phase of the interview termed

    A. introductory.

    B. ongoing.

    C. working.

    D. closure.

_____ 3. The nurse is preparing to interview an adult client for the first time. The nurse observes that the client appears very anxious. The nurse should

    A. allow the client time to calm down.

    B. avoid discussing sensitive issues.

    C. set time limits with the client.

    D. explain the role and purpose of the nurse.

_____ 4. The nurse is beginning a health history interview with an adult client who expresses anger at the nurse. The best approach for dealing with an angry client is for the nurse to

    A. allow the client to ventilate his or her feelings.

    B. offer reasons why the client shouldn't feel angry.

    C. provide structure during the interview.

    D. refer the client to a different health care provider.

_____ 5. The nurse is planning to interview a client who is being treated for depression. When the nurse enters the examination room, the client is sitting on the table with shoulders slumped. The nurse should plan to approach this client by

    A. providing the client with simple explanations.

    B. offering to hold the client's hand.

    C. using a highly structured interview process.

    D. expressing interest in a neutral manner.

_____ 6. The nurse is planning to interview a client who has demonstrated manipulative behaviors during past clinic visits. During the interview process, the nurse should plan to

    A. give the client rules with which he must agree to comply.

    B. provide structure and set limits with the client.

    C. tell the client that the nurse is aware of his past behaviors.

    D. approach the client in an authoritative manner.

_____ 7. During a client interview, the nurse asks questions about the client's past health history. The primary purpose of asking about past health problems is to

    A. determine whether genetic conditions are present.

    B. summarize the family's health problems.

    C. evaluate how the client's current symptoms affect lifestyle.

    D. identify risk factors to the client and his or her significant others.

_____ 8. While interviewing an adult client about her nutrition habits, the nurse should

    A. ask the client for a three-day recall of food intake.

    B. review the food pyramid with the client.

    C. ask the client about limitations to activity.

    D. encourage the client to drink three to four glasses of water daily.

_____ 9. While interviewing an adult client about the client's stress levels and coping responses, an appropriate question by the nurse is

    A. "Do you feel stress at work?"

    B. "How often do you feel stressed?"

    C. "Is stress a problem in your life?"

    D. "How do you manage your stress?"

MATCHING

Match the terms in the left column with the correct description in the right column.

Term	Description
_____ 1. Biographical data	A. Sunburns easily; occasional headaches; no breathing problems or problems with heart; breast soreness before menstruation; found lump in right breast while doing BSE; no problems with circulation; no complaints of stiff joints or sore muscles; no dizziness, confusion, or forgetfulness
_____ 2. Reason for seeking healthcare	
_____ 3. History of present concern	
	B. No previous problems; occasional breast soreness before menstruation
_____ 4. Past health history	
_____ 5. Family health history	C. Exercises three times a week; drinks "a lot" of caffeine to keep alert and on the go for long, busy days; high stress (from work); good relationships with husband and children
_____ 6. Review of body systems for current health problem	
	D. Felt lump in right breast while doing BSE
	E. Middlescent: generativity vs. stagnation
_____ 7. Lifestyle and health practices	F. Great-aunt had breast cancer; sister has fibrocystic breast disease
	G. Female client; aged 42; married; two children
_____ 8. Developmental level	H. All childhood diseases; one hospitalization to set a badly broken arm (car accident); two normal vaginal deliveries

■ Self-Reflection and Evaluation of Learner Objectives

After reading Chapter 4 in the text and completing the above exercises, please identify to what degree you have met each of the following chapter learning objectives. For those objectives that you have met partially or not at all, you will want to review chapter content for that learning objective.

Objective	Very much	Somewhat	Not at all

INTERVIEWING

1. Describe the three phases of the interview.
2. Describe the use of nonverbal communication during the interview.
3. Describe the use of effective verbal communication during a client interview.
4. Describe types of verbal communication that should be avoided in client interviews.
5. Describe how communication should be varied to communicate with elderly clients.
6. Describe how ethnicity can affect communication.
7. Describe appropriate ways to modify communication with clients who have emotional conditions.

TAKING THE HEALTH HISTORY

1. Identify the major categories of a complete health history.
2. Describe key sources of biographical data.
3. Describe types of biographical data to be collected.
4. Obtain an accurate nursing history of a client, omitting (at this time) the review of body systems.
5. Use the SWIPE format to collect information about a health concern.
6. Construct a genogram to identify patterns within family history.
7. Identify information to be obtained in a review of body systems.
8. Describe the relationship of the lifestyle and health practices profile to health status.
9. Compare data obtained in a health history with normal developmental parameters for a client.

For additional information on this book, be sure to visit *http://connection.lww.com.*

Collecting Objective Data

CHAPTER OVERVIEW

The pages of this chapter can help you review the reasons and techniques for obtaining objective assessment data (data that are observable and/or measurable).

■ Chapter Pretest

MATCHING

Match the terms in the left column with the correct description in the right column.

Term	Description
_____ 1. Sims' position	A. Part of examiner's hand used to feel for temperature
_____ 2. Sitting position	B. Side-lying position used during the rectal examination
_____ 3. Supine position	C. Position used during much of the physical examination, including examination of the head, neck, lungs, chest, back, breast, axilla, heart, vital signs, and upper extremities
_____ 4. Standing position	
_____ 5. Prone position	
_____ 6. Lithotomy position	D. Back-lying position used for examination of the abdomen (with small pillow under head and one under knees). This position also allows easy access for palpatation of peripheral pulses
_____ 7. Fingerpads	
_____ 8. Ulnar surface or palm of hand	E. Larger end of stethoscope used to detect breath sounds, normal heart sounds, and bowel sounds
_____ 9. Dorsal surface of hand	F. Position used to examine male genitalia and to assess gait, posture, and balance
_____ 10. Bell of stethoscope	
_____ 11. Diaphragm of stethoscope	G. Part of examiner's hand used to feel for fine discriminations: pulses, texture, size, consistency, shape, and crepitus
	H. Client lies on abdomen with head turned to side; may be used to assess back and mobility of hip joint
	I. Part of examiner's hand used to feel for vibration, thrills, or fremitus
	J. Smaller end of stethoscope used to detect low-pitched sounds (abnormal heart sounds and bruits)
	K. Back-lying position with hips at edge of examining table and feet supported in stirrups; used for examination of female genitalia, reproductive tract, and rectum

■ Learner Activities

After reading Chapter 5, participate in the following activities with your lab partner as assigned.

WORKING WITH PEERS IN LEARNING LAB

1. Recall a time when you were about to have a physical examination. Remember the anxieties and concerns you were feeling. What were your greatest fears? Share these feelings with your lab partner.

2. Now practice verbally preparing your lab partner for a physical examination. Explain privacy, confidentiality, time, positioning, and the purpose of the examination.

3. Inspect the forearm of your lab partner. Do you have sufficient lighting? Explain. Now use Table 5-2 in the textbook to use various parts of your hand to palpate pulses, texture, shape, and temperature of the forearm.

4. Practice indirect percussion (see Fig. 5-6) on your lab partner to determine the various percussion tones listed in Table 5-3. Use studs in walls to percuss flat and dull tones. Fill a milk carton part way with water and percuss it. Percuss an empty milk carton and notice the difference. What different types of percussion notes are you hearing?

5. Read Display 5-3 on "How to Use a Stethoscope." Discuss with your lab partner whether this is how you normally use a stethoscope. What did you learn?

6. Use Table 5-1, "Equipment Needed for a Physical Examination," to identify the equipment pieces needed. Find each of these pieces of equipment in your learning lab, and discuss its purpose and how to use it with your lab partner.

■ Chapter Post-test

MULTIPLE CHOICE

Choose one best answer for each of the following multiple-choice questions.

_____ 1. Before beginning a physical assessment of a client, the nurse should first
   A. wash both hands with soap and water.
   B. determine whether the client is anxious.
   C. ask the client to remove all clothing.
   D. request a family member to be present.

_____ 2. To alleviate a client's anxiety during a comprehensive assessment, the nurse should
   A. begin with intrusive procedures first to get them completed quickly.
   B. explain each procedure being performed and the reason for the procedure.

C. remain in the examination room while the client changes into a gown.

D. ask the client to sign a consent for the physical examination.

_____ 3. While performing a physical examination on an older adult, the nurse should plan to

A. complete the examination as quickly as possible.

B. ask the client to change positions frequently.

C. provide only minimal teaching related to health care.

D. use minimal position changes during the examination.

_____ 4. During a comprehensive assessment, the primary technique used by the nurse throughout the examination is

A. palpation.

B. percussion.

C. auscultation.

D. inspection.

_____ 5. While examining a client, the nurse plans to palpate temperature of the skin by using the

A. fingertips of the hand.

B. ulnar surface of the hand.

C. dorsal surface of the hand.

D. palmar surface of the hand.

_____ 6. During palpation of the client's organs, the nurse palpates the spleen by applying pressure between 2.5 and 5 centimeters. The nurse is performing

A. light palpation.

B. moderate palpation.

C. deep palpation.

D. very deep palpation.

_____ 7. While performing a physical examination on an adult client, the nurse can detect the density of an underlying structure by using

A. inspection.

B. palpation.

C. Doppler magnification.

D. percussion.

_____ 8. When the nurse places one hand flat on the body surface and uses the fist of the other hand to strike the back of the hand flat on the body surface, the nurse is using

A. firm percussion.

B. direct percussion.

C. indirect percussion.

D. blunt percussion.

_____ 9. An adult client visits the clinic and tells the nurse that she suspects she has a urinary tract infection. In order to detect tenderness over the client's kidneys, the nurse should instruct the client that the nurse will be performing

   A. moderate palpation.

   B. deep palpation.

   C. indirect percussion.

   D. blunt percussion.

_____ 10. The most commonly used method of percussion is

   A. direct percussion.

   B. mild percussion.

   C. indirect percussion.

   D. blunt percussion.

_____ 11. During a comprehensive assessment of the lungs of an adult client with a diagnosis of emphysema, the nurse anticipates that during percussion the client will exhibit

   A. hyperresonance.

   B. tympany.

   C. dullness.

   D. flatness

_____ 12. While percussing an adult client during a physical examination, the nurse can expect to hear flatness over the client's

   A. lungs.

   B. bone.

   C. liver.

   D. abdomen.

_____ 13. During a comprehensive assessment of an adult client, the nurse can best hear high-pitched sounds by using a stethoscope with a

   A. 1-inch bell.

   B. 1 1/2-inch diaphragm.

   C. 15-inch flexible tubing.

   D. 1-inch diaphragm.

ESSAY QUESTIONS

1. When might you use deep palpation during a physical examination? Bimanual palpation? Direct percussion? Indirect percussion?

2. Explain how the universal precautions and infection control guidelines would apply to the physical examination techniques of inspection, percussion, palpation, and auscultation.

3. Describe how you would prepare yourself to perform a total physical examination of a client of the opposite sex. Describe how you would prepare the client both emotionally and physically.

■ Self-Reflection and Evaluation of Learner Objectives

After reading Chapter 5 in the text and completing the above reviews, please identify to what degree you have met each of the following chapter learning objectives. For those objectives that you have met partially or not at all, you will want to review chapter content for that learning objective.

Objective	Very much	Somewhat	Not at all
1. Describe ways to prepare the physical environment and make it conducive to a physical examination.			
2. Explain ways to prepare the client for a physical examination.			
3. Describe the various positions used to perform the physical examination.			
4. Demonstrate the correct method used for inspection during the physical examination.			
5. Explain the purpose and differences between light, deep, and bimanual palpation.			
6. Demonstrate correct direct, indirect, and blunt percussion techniques used during the physical examination.			
7. Explain the correct use of the stethoscope and the purpose of the bell and the diaphragm.			
8. Survey the various pieces of equipment used to perform a physical examination.			

For additional information on this book, be sure to visit *http://connection.lww.com.*

Validating and Documenting Data

CHAPTER OVERVIEW

After you collect assessment data, what do you do with them? How do you know that they are reliable information? How do they become part of the client's record? Use the following activities to review and enhance the validation and documentation process.

■ Chapter Pretest

MULTIPLE CHOICE

Choose one best answer for each of the following multiple-choice questions.

_____ 1. If the nurse makes an error while documenting findings on a client's record, the nurse should

   A. erase the error and make the correction.

   B. obliterate the error and make the correction.

   C. draw a line through the error and have it witnessed.

   D. draw a line through the error, writing "error," and initialing.

_____ 2. The nurse is preparing to document assessment findings in a client's record. The nurse should

   A. write in complete sentences with few abbreviations.

   B. avoid slang terms or labels unless they are direct quotes.

   C. record how the data were collected.

   D. use the term *normal* for normal findings.

_____ 3. The nurse has assessed the breath sounds of an adult client. The best way for the nurse to document these findings on a client is to write

   A. "Bilateral lung sounds clear."

   B. "The client's lung sounds were clear on both sides."

   C. "Client's lung sounds were auscultated with stethoscope and were clear on both sides."

   D. "After listening to client's lung sounds, both lungs appeared clear."

_____ 4. An example of an objective finding in an adult client is

   A. a client's symptom of pain.

   B. family history data.

   C. genetic disorders.

   D. vital signs.

_____ 5. While recording the subjective data of an adult client who complains of pain in his lower back, the nurse should include the location of the pain and the

A. cause of the pain.

B. client's caregiver.

C. client's occupation.

D. pain relief measures.

_____ 6. One disadvantage of the open-ended assessment form is that it

A. doesn't allow for individualization.

B. asks standardized questions.

C. requires a lot of time to complete.

D. doesn't provide a total picture of the client.

_____ 7. The nurse is recording admission data for an adult client using a cued or checklist type of assessment form. This type of assessment form

A. prevents missed questions during data collection.

B. covers all the data that a client may provide.

C. clusters the assessment data with nursing diagnoses.

D. establishes comparability of data across populations.

_____ 8. One advantage for an institution to use an integrated cued/checklist type of assessment data form is that it

A. allows a comprehensive and thorough picture of the client's symptoms.

B. may be easily used by different levels of caregivers, which enhances communication.

C. provides for easy and rapid documentation across clinical settings and populations.

D. includes the 11 health care patterns in an easily readable format.

_____ 9. An assessment form commonly used in long-term care facilities is the nursing minimum data set. One primary advantage to this type of assessment form is that it

A. establishes comparability of nursing data across clinical populations.

B. clusters all of the nursing and medical diagnoses in one place.

C. allows for individualization for each client in the health care setting.

D. uses a flow chart format for easy documentation of objective data.

_____ 10. In some health care settings, the institution uses an assessment form that assesses only one part of a client. These types of forms are termed

A. progressive.

B. specific.

C. checklist.

D. focused.

_____ 11. The nurse is planning to assess a newly admitted adult client. While gathering data from the client, the nurse should

    A. validate all data before documentation of the data.

    B. document the data after the entire examination process.

    C. record the nurse's understanding of the client's problem.

    D. use medical terms that are commonly used in health care settings.

LEARNER ACTIVITIES

After reading Chapter 6 in the text, participate in the following activities with your lab partner as assigned.

1. Select a case from the end of one of the body systems chapters in the textbook (e.g., Chapter 9 or Chapter 10) and read it. Separate the objective from the subjective data. Now determine what data need to be validated. How would you validate them?

2. Interview your lab partner to determine how his or her physical and mental health has been during the past month. Do this by beginning with five basic questions:

    a. How have you felt during the past month?

    b. Have you had any major illnesses during this time?

    c. Have you had any minor illnesses during this time?

    d. Rate your current health on a scale of 1 to 10 (with 1 being poor and 10 being great).

    e. How would you like your health to improve?

■ Chapter Post-test

MATCHING

Match the following items with either subjective (S) or objective (O) DATA.

1. Describes severe right-sided headache

2. Reddened, raised, indurated area on deltoid area of left arm

3. Cannot eat seeds or uncooked grains without abdominal discomfort

4. Passing flatus

5. Bowel sounds present in all four quadrants

6. Complains of lower back pain on movement

7. Pattern of request for pain medication every two hours

8. Pale, clammy, and diaphoretic

9. Feels nauseated and dizzy

10. Emesis of 200 mL light beige thin liquid

ESSAY QUESTIONS

1. Discuss the possible results of failing to document data. How could this affect the client? The nurse?

2. Discuss a variety of ways to validate client data obtained during a nursing history interview.

3. Document narrative progress notes on the following client information, adding hypothetical details as needed for a complete entry.

   Mrs. Jones arrives in room 2344. Headache; flushed, cool skin; pale; nausea and vomiting; temperature normal; blood pressure 136/85 mm Hg; pulse rapid; respirations rapid. Requesting pain medication.

■ Self-Reflection and Evaluation of Learner Objectives

After reading Chapter 6 in the text and completing the above reviews, please identify to what degree you have met each of the following chapter learning objectives. For those objectives that you have met partially or not at all, you will want to review chapter content for that learning objective.

Objective	Very much	Somewhat	Not at all
1. Define validation of data.			
2. Describe the steps of the validation process.			
3. Describe conditions that require data to be rechecked and validated.			
4. Discuss several ways to validate data.			
5. Describe the purposes of documenting assessment data.			
6. Describe the general guidelines and rules for documenting data.			
7. Describe the three types of standardized assessment forms for documenting data.			
8. Document assessment findings, using a variety of assessment forms (e.g., narrative progress notes, flow sheets).			
9. Discuss the significance of documentation as specified by your state nurse practice act and JCAHO standards.			

For additional information on this book, be sure to visit *http://connection.lww.com.*

Using Diagnostic Reasoning Skills to Analyze Data

CHAPTER OVERVIEW

Initially, sorting through nursing assessment data may seem to be an overwhelming task. Use the exercises that follow to divide the process known as diagnostic reasoning into doable components. Use the activities to review the steps of critical thinking and diagnostic reasoning, to differentiate normal findings from abnormal findings, to draw inferences, to make nursing diagnoses, and to confirm or rule out conclusions.

■ Chapter Pretest

MATCHING

Match the terms in the left column with the correct description in the right column.

Term	Description
_____ 1. Critical thinking	A. A nursing diagnosis that indicates the client has an opportunity for enhancement of a health status
_____ 2. Intuition	B. Certain physiologic complications that nurses monitor to detect their onset or change in status
_____ 3. Wellness nursing diagnosis	
_____ 4. Collaborative problem	C. Aptitude involving the act or process of knowing, including both awareness and judgment
_____ 5. Risk nursing diagnosis	D. The fact or condition of knowing something with familiarity gained through experience or association
_____ 6. Actual nursing diagnosis	E. Quick and ready insight
_____ 7. Knowledge	F. The way in which one processes information using knowledge, past experience, intuition, and cognitive abilities in order to formulate conclusions or diagnoses
_____ 8. Cognitive abilities	
_____ 9. Analysis of data	G. Diagnostic phase of the nursing process
	H. A nursing diagnosis that indicates the client does not currently have a problem but is at high risk for developing it
	I. A nursing diagnosis that indicates the client is currently experiencing the stated problem or has a dysfunctional pattern

■ Chapter Post-test

MULTIPLE CHOICE

Choose one best answer for each of the following multiple-choice questions.

_____ 1. One characteristic of a nurse who is a critical thinker is the ability to

    A. form an opinion quickly.

    B. offer advice to clients.

    C. be right most of the time.

    D. validate information and judgments.

_____ 2. Before the nurse analyzes the data collected, the nurse should

    A. determine collaborative problems with the health care team.

    B. group the data into clusters or groups of problems.

    C. generate possible hypotheses for the client's problems.

    D. perform the steps of the assessment process accurately.

_____ 3. The nurse is caring for an adult client who tells the nurse "For weeks now, I just can't get to sleep at night because of all the noise in my neighborhood." An actual nursing diagnosis for this client is

    A. fatigue related to excessive noise levels as manifested by client's statements of chronic fatigue.

    B. sleep deprivation related to noisy neighborhood and inability to sleep.

    C. chronic fatigue syndrome related to excessive levels of noise in neighborhood.

    D. opportunity to enhance sleep related to control of noise level in the home.

_____ 4. A common error for beginning nurses who are formulating nursing diagnoses during data analysis is to

    A. formulate too many nursing diagnoses for the client and family.

    B. include too much data about the client in the history.

    C. obtain an insufficient number of cues and cluster patterns.

    D. quickly make a diagnosis without hypothesizing several diagnoses.

■ Learner Activities

After reading Chapter 7 in the text , participate in the following activities with your lab partner as assigned.

1. Refer to the first page of Chapter 7 and ask yourself the 10 questions presented to determine your level of critical thinking. Discuss with your peers ways to improve your critical thinking based on these questions.

2. Interview your lab partners to assess their current level of well-being for the day. Use the seven steps for analyzing data to draw conclusions. Can you identify any nursing diagnoses or collaborative problems?

3. Review the diagnostic reasoning pitfalls in Chapter 7. Discuss with your partners which pitfalls you feel you will make most frequently. How will experience help you to avoid these pitfalls?

■ Chapter Post-test

ESSAY QUESTIONS

1. Discuss how critical thinking is used in the assessment phase of the nursing process.

2. Describe the steps you go through to draw conclusions from gathered data.

3. Read the following case study. Identify a cue cluster and possible diagnostic conclusion(s) (wellness, risk, or actual nursing diagnosis). Describe your critical thinking process.

Mrs. Phillips has smoked three packs of cigarettes a day for 50 years. She complains of difficulty fixing her own meals and bathing and dressing herself because of fatigue and shortness of breath. She has a nonproductive congested-sounding cough, a respiratory rate of 26 beats/minute, a shallow breathing pattern, an oral temperature of 97.8 degrees F, and a blood pressure of 140/92 mm Hg. Height 5 feet, 3 inches; weight 127 pounds.

■ Self-Reflection and Evaluation of Learner Objectives

After reading Chapter 7 in the text and completing the above reviews, please identify to what degree you have met each of the following chapter learning objectives. For those objectives that you have met partially or not at all, you will want to review chapter content for that learning objective.

Objective	Very much	Somewhat	Not at all
1. Describe how critical thinking relates to diagnostic reasoning.			
2. Determine your own ability to think critically.			
3. Describe seven essential critical thinking characteristics.			
4. List the six essential components of the diagnostic phase of the nursing process.			
5. List the seven distinct steps used in this text to perform data analysis.			
6. Describe and give examples of wellness, risk, and actual nursing diagnoses.			
7. Give examples of collaborative problems.			
8. Explain why experienced, expert nurses have an advantage over novice nurses in making accurate diagnoses.			
9. Describe diagnostic reasoning pitfalls.			

For additional information on this book, be sure to visit *http://connection.lww.com*.

UNIT II

Nursing Assessment of the Adult

CHAPTER 8

General Survey and Nutritional Assessment

CHAPTER OVERVIEW

Your initial impression of the client, his or her vital signs, and his or her nutritional status combine to give you a starting point for assessing the client's general health condition. The following exercises and quizzes can help you review the basics.

■ Chapter Pretest

MULTIPLE CHOICE

Choose one best answer for each of the following multiple-choice questions.

_____ 1. The nurse is preparing to assess an adult client in the clinic. The nurse observes that the client is wearing lightweight clothing although the temperature is below freezing outside. The nurse anticipates that the client may be

    A. abusing drugs.

    B. a victim of abuse.

    C. poor.

    D. anxious.

_____ 2. An elderly client is seen by the nurse in the neighborhood clinic. The nurse observes that the client is dressed in several layers of clothing, although the temperature is warm outside. The nurse suspects that the client's cold intolerance is a result of

    A. decreased body metabolism.

    B. neurologic deficits.

    C. recent surgery.

    D. pancreatic disease.

MATCHING

Match the terms in the left column with the correct description in the right column.

Term	Description
_____ 1. 36.5 to 37.0°C (96.0 to 99.9°F)	A. Normal diastolic blood pressure range
_____ 2. 60 to 100 beats per minute	B. Diastolic blood pressure
_____ 3. 12 to 20 per minute	C. Normal oral temperature
_____ 4. Highest pressure exerted on artery walls	D. Normal systolic blood pressure range
_____ 5. Lowest pressure exerted on artery walls	E. Normal respiratory rate
_____ 6. Difference between systolic and diastolic pressure	F. Normal pulse
_____ 7. 100 to 140 mm Hg	G. Systolic blood pressure
_____ 8. 60 to 90 mm Hg	H. Pulse pressure

■ Learner Activities

1. Go a public place, such as a store or a shopping mall, and practice observing passersby. Look for general characteristics of physical and sexual development. Observe color, dress, hygiene, posture and gait, body build, consciousness level, comfort level, behavior, facial expression, and speech.

2. Practice taking vital signs and anthropometric measurements on peers, friends, and family members. Try to find a variety of people: obese, thin, elderly, young. Practice recording your findings on flow charts.

PERFORMING PHYSICAL ASSESSMENT

Practice recording general survey findings. Use the following Physical Assessment Checklist to assess a peer, friend, or family member.

PHYSICAL ASSESSMENT CHECKLIST

Assessment Skill	Findings (Normal or Abnormal) and Notes		Performance (Satisfactory, Needs Improvement, Unsatisfactory)		
	N	A	S	N	U
Impression of the Client					
1. Observe physical development (appears to be chronologic age) and sexual development (appropriate for gender and age).	☐	☐	☐	☐	☐
2. Observe skin (generalized color, color variation, and condition).	☐	☐	☐	☐	☐
3. Observe dress (occasion and weather appropriate).	☐	☐	☐	☐	☐
4. Observe hygiene (cleanliness, odor, grooming).	☐	☐	☐	☐	☐

PHYSICAL ASSESSMENT CHECKLIST

Assessment Skill	Findings (Normal or Abnormal) and Notes		Performance (Satisfactory, Needs Improvement, Unsatisfactory)		
	N	A	S	N	U
5. Observe posture (erect and comfortable) and gait (rhythmic and coordinated).	☐	☐	☐	☐	☐
6. Observe body build (muscle mass and fat distribution).	☐	☐	☐	☐	☐
7. Observe consciousness level (alertness, orientation, appropriateness).	☐	☐	☐	☐	☐
8. Observe comfort level.	☐	☐	☐	☐	☐
9. Observe behavior (body movements, affect, cooperativeness, purposefulness, and appropriateness).	☐	☐	☐	☐	☐
10. Observe facial expression (culture-appropriate eye contact and facial expression).	☐	☐	☐	☐	☐
11. Observe speech (pattern and style).	☐	☐	☐	☐	☐
Vital Signs					
1. Gather equipment (thermometer, sphygmomanometer, stethoscope, and watch).	☐	☐	☐	☐	☐
2. Measure temperature (oral, axillary, rectal, tympanic).	☐	☐	☐	☐	☐
3. Measure radial pulse (rate, rhythm, amplitude and contour, and elasticity).	☐	☐	☐	☐	☐
4. Monitor respirations (rate, rhythm, and depth).	☐	☐	☐	☐	☐
5. Measure blood pressure.					
Antropometric Measurements					
1. Gather equipment (balance beam scale with height attachment, metric measuring tape, marking pencil, and skinfold calipers).	☐	☐	☐	☐	☐
2. Measure height.	☐	☐	☐	☐	☐
3. Calculate frame size (r = height/wrist circumference).	☐	☐	☐	☐	☐
4. Measure weight (desirable weights table, p. 90 (1 lb = 2.205 kg).	☐	☐	☐	☐	☐
5. Determine ideal body weight (IBW) using formula on page 102.	☐	☐	☐	☐	☐
6. Calculate percentage of ideal body weight (% IBW = actual weight/IBW × 100).	☐	☐	☐	☐	☐
7. Measure body mass index (BMI) (BMI = weight in kilograms/height in meters).	☐	☐	☐	☐	☐
8. Determine waist-to-hip ratio (waist-to-hip ratio = waist circumference/hip circumference).	☐	☐	☐	☐	☐
9. Measure mid-arm circumference (MAC) as described on page 103 and compare with tables on page 109.	☐	☐	☐	☐	☐
10. Measure triceps skinfold thickness (TSF) as described on page 104 and compare with tables on page 109.	☐	☐	☐	☐	☐

(continues)

PHYSICAL ASSESSMENT CHECKLIST *(Continued)*

Assessment Skill	Findings (Normal or Abnormal) and Notes		Performance (Satisfactory, Needs Improvement, Unsatisfactory)		
	N	A	S	N	U
11. Calculate mid-arm muscle circumference (MAMC). (MAMC (cm) = MAC (cm) – [0.314 × TSF]).	☐	☐	☐	☐	☐
Analysis of Data					
1. Formulate nursing diagnoses (wellness, risk, actual).	☐	☐	☐	☐	☐
2. Formulate collaborative problems.	☐	☐	☐	☐	☐
3. Make necessary referrals.	☐	☐	☐	☐	☐

CASE STUDY

On the basis of the following case study assessment information, work through the steps of analyzing the data. Identify abnormal data and strengths in **subjective and objective findings,** assemble **cue clusters,** draw **inferences,** make possible **nursing diagnoses,** identify **defining characteristics, confirm or rule out** the diagnoses, and **document** your conclusions. Use the blank diagnostic analysis charts provided at the end of this book to guide your thinking. You may want to write on the chart or use separate paper. In either case, propose nursing diagnoses that are specific to the client in the case study. Identify collaborative problems, if any, for this client. Finally, identify data, if any, that point toward a medical problem requiring a referral.

Steve Martin is a 36-year-old Caucasian man who comes to the employee health center for advice. He says he has been under a lot of stress lately. He believes he is drinking too much coffee (12 cups daily) and smoking more than usual (2 packs daily). He is neatly and appropriately dressed in a business suit. His posture is erect, and his gait is smooth. His hands are trembling. He has excess subcutaneous fat, distributed primarily around the waist. Mr. Martin appears tired, anxious, and hurried. He is cooperative, maintains good eye contact, and answers questions quickly. His speech is clear and fast paced.

Vital Signs

Oral temperature: 98.6 degrees F
Radial pulse: 92 beats/minute, strong but irregular
Respirations: 23 breaths/minute, shallow, and somewhat labored
Blood pressure: sitting, right arm 160/110 mm Hg, left arm 162/112 mm Hg; standing, 155/100 mm Hg (standing BP taken in either arm due to similarity of sitting BPs)

Anthropometric Measurements

Height: 5 feet 10 inches
Weight: 203 pounds
MAC: 32.3
TSF: 14.1
MAMC: 25.7

■ Chapter Post-test

MULTIPLE CHOICE

Choose one best answer for each of the following multiple-choice questions.

_____ 1. The nurse is assessing an elderly postsurgical client in the home. To begin the physical examination, the nurse should first assess the client's

A. height and weight.

B. ability to swallow.

C. vital signs.

D. gait.

_____ 2. While caring for an 80-year-old client in his home, the nurse determines that the client's temperature is 96.5 degrees F. The nurse determines that the client is most likely exhibiting

A. normal changes that occur with the aging process.

B. hypothermia that occurs before an infectious process.

C. a metabolic disorder resulting in circulatory changes.

D. an immune disorder resulting in low platelet count.

_____ 3. The nurse is preparing to assess the respirations of an alert adult client. The nurse should

A. explain to the client that he or she will be counting the client's respirations.

B. observe for equal bilateral chest expansion of 1 to 2 inches.

C. count for 15 seconds and multiply the number by four to obtain the rate.

D. ask the client to lie in a supine position, which makes counting the respirations easier.

_____ 4. While assessing an older adult client's respirations, the nurse can anticipate that the respiratory pattern may exhibit a

A. shorter inspiratory phase.

B. longer inspiratory phase.

C. shorter expiratory phase.

D. longer expiratory phase.

_____ 5. The nurse is caring for a client who is having nothing by mouth (NPO) on the first postoperative day. The client's blood pressure was 120/80 mm Hg approximately four hours ago, but it is now 140/88 mm Hg. The nurse should ask the client

A. "Are you taking any medications for hypertension?"

B. "Do you have enough blankets to stay warm?"

C. "Are you having pain from your surgery?"

D. "What is your typical blood pressure reading?"

_____ 6. A normal pulse pressure range for an adult client is typically

A. 20 to 40 mm Hg.

B. 30 to 50 mm Hg.

    C. 40 to 60 mm Hg.

    D. 60 to 80 mm Hg.

_____ 7. The nurse determines that a 45-year-old male client with a medium frame who is 5 feet 10 inches tall weighs 210 pounds. He tells the nurse that he "eats well, but doesn't do much exercise because of a foot ailment." An appropriate nursing diagnosis for this client is

    A. normal body nutrition related to healthy eating patterns.

    B. altered body nutrition: less than body requirements.

    C. obesity related to lack of exercise because of foot ailment.

    D. imbalanced body nutrition: more than body requirements.

_____ 8. The nurse is caring for an adult female client whose waist-to-hip ratio is greater than 0.80. The nurse should instruct the client that she is at greater risk for

    A. heart attack.

    B. ovarian cancer.

    C. stomach cancer.

    D. osteoporosis.

_____ 9. The nurse is preparing to measure the triceps skinfold of an adult client. The nurse should

    A. ask the client to assume a sitting position.

    B. measure the triceps skinfold in the dominant arm.

    C. pull the skin toward the muscle mass of the arm.

    D. repeat the procedure three times and average the measurements.

■ Self-Reflection and Evaluation of Learner Objectives

After reading Chapter 8 in the text and completing the above reviews, please identify to what degree you have met each of the following chapter learning objectives. For those objectives that you have met partially or not at all, you will want to review chapter content for that objective.

Objective	Very much	Somewhat	Not at all
1. Describe the three parts of the general survey.			
2. Explain how to prepare the client for the first segment of the general survey.			
3. Assess the client's physical and sexual development.			
4. Assess the overall appearance and color of the skin; the type of clothing the client is wearing; and the client's hygiene, posture, gait, body build, muscle mass, and fat distribution.			

Objective	Very much	Somewhat	Not at all
5. Assess level of consciousness, comfort level, and behavior; facial expression for eye contact and appropriate smiling and frowning; and speech style and pattern.			
6. Obtain accurate vital signs as part of the general survey			
7. Identify and explain how to use the equipment needed to obtain vital signs and temperature.			
8. Describe temperature variations in the older adult.			
9. Discuss how to obtain accurate measurement of the radial and apical pulses.			
10. Obtain an accurate respiratory rate, and describe expected changes that may be apparent in the assessment of an older client's pulse, respiratory rate, and blood pressure.			
11. Obtain an accurate measurement of blood pressure, and discuss the parameters for blood pressure (normal as well as the four stages of hypertension)			
12. Assess for orthostatic (postural) hypotension if the client is taking antihypertensive drugs or has a history of fainting or dizziness.			
13. Describe the equipment needed to perform anthropometric measurement, and obtain accurate measurements (height, frame size, weight, body mass index, waist-to-hip ratio, mid-arm circumference, triceps skinfold thickness, and mid-arm muscle circumference).			
14. Describe expected changes with height and weight associated with the aging process.			
15. Calculate frame size, determine a client's ideal body weight (IBW), and calculate the client's percentage of ideal body weight along with body mass index (BMI).			
16. Explain the importance of waist-to-hip ratio, mid-arm circumference, triceps skinfold thickness, midarm muscle circumference.			
17. Discuss possible nursing diagnoses and collaborative problems that may emerge after a general survey.			

For additional information on this book, be sure to visit *http://connection.lww.com*.

Skin, Hair, and Nail Assessment

CHAPTER OVERVIEW

In any kind of nursing assessment, the client's skin, hair, and nails are among the most easily observed characteristics. They also provide clues to the client's general health condition. The following questions and exercise are presented to help you review your observation and other assessment skills. You will also be helped, both in your studies and in your practice, by the directions for performing a skin self-assessment, which may be found at the end of this chapter.

■ Chapter Pretest

MULTIPLE CHOICE

Choose the one best answer for each of the following multiple-choice questions.

_____ 1. Connecting the skin to underlying structures is/are the
   A. papillae.
   B. sebaceous glands.
   C. dermis layer.
   D. subcutaneous tissue.

_____ 2. The skin plays a vital role in temperature maintenance, fluid and electrolyte balance, and synthesis of vitamin
   A. A.
   B. B_{12}.
   C. C.
   D. D.

_____ 3. The only layer of the skin that undergoes cell division is the
   A. innermost layer of the epidermis.
   B. outermost layer of the epidermis.
   C. innermost layer of the dermis.
   D. outermost layer of the dermis.

_____ 4. A client's skin color depends on melanin and carotene contained in the skin, and the
   A. client's genetic background.
   B. volume of blood circulating in the dermis.
   C. number of lymph vessels near the dermis.
   D. vascularity of the apocrine glands.

_____ 5. Hair follicles, sebaceous glands, and sweat glands originate from the
   A. epidermis.
   B. eccrine glands.
   C. keratinized tissue.
   D. dermis.

_____ 6. The apocrine glands are dormant until puberty and are concentrated in the axillae, the perineum, and the
   A. areola of the breast.
   B. entire skin surface.
   C. soles of the feet.
   D. adipose tissue.

_____ 7. Short, pale, and fine hair that is present over much of the body is termed
   A. vellus.
   B. dermal.
   C. lanugo.
   D. terminal.

_____ 8. A primary function of hair in the nose and eyelashes is to serve as a
   A. response to cold.
   B. filter for dust.
   C. pigment producer.
   D. response to fright.

_____ 9. The nails, located on the distal phalanges of the fingers and toes, are composed of
   A. ectodermal cells.
   B. endodermal cells.
   C. keratinized epidermal cells.
   D. stratum cells.

■ Labeling Activities

Label the following skin structures.

Skin and hair follicles and related structures.

Label the structure indicated by the line; then match your answer with the label on the matching figure in chapter 9 of your textbook.

Label the following nail structures.

Nails and related structures.

Label the structure indicated by the line; then match your answer with the label on the matching figure in chapter 9 of your textbook.

■ Learner Activities

WORKING WITH PEERS IN LEARNING LAB

1. Review the information in Display 9-1. Then, determine your own risk for skin cancer. Next, identify and discuss ethnic groups that are at highest risk for skin cancer.

DISPLAY 9-1. **How to Examine Your Own Skin**

You can systematically and regularly assess your skin for abnormalities by using the following recommended procedure for skin assessment from the American Cancer Society.

Step 1

Make sure the room is well-lighted, and that you have nearby a full-length mirror, a hand-held mirror, a hand-held blow dryer, and two chairs or stools. Undress completely.

Step 2

Hold your hands with the palms face up, as shown in the drawing. Look at your palms, fingers, spaces between the fingers, and forearms. Then turn your hands over and examine the backs of your hands, fingers, spaces between the fingers, fingernails, and forearms.

Step 3

Now position yourself in front of the full-length mirror. Hold up your arms, bent at the elbows, with your palms facing you. In the mirror, look at the backs of your forearms and elbows.

Step 4

Again, using the full-length mirror, observe the enitre front of your body. In turn, look at your face, neck, and arms. Turn your palms to face the mirror and look at your upper arms. Then look at your chest and abdomen; pubic area; thighs and lower legs.

Step 5

Still standing in front of the mirror, lift your arms over your head with the palms facing each other. Turn so that your right side is facing the mirror and look at the entire side of your body: your hands and arms, underarms, sides of your trunk, thighs, and lower legs. Then turn, and repeat the process with your left side.

Step 6

With your back toward the full-length mirror, look at your buttocks and the back of your thighs and lower legs.

Step 7

Now pick up the hand-held mirror. With your back still to the full-length mirror, examine the back of your neck, and your back and buttocks. Also examine the backs of your arms in this way. Some areas are hard to see, and you may find it helpful to ask your spouse or a friend to assist you.

Step 8

Use the hand-held mirror and the full-length mirror to look at your scalp. Because the scalp is difficult to examine, we suggest you use a hand-held blow dryer turned to a cool setting, to lift the hair from the scalp. While some people find it easy to hold the mirror in one hand and the dryer in the other while looking in the full-length mirror, many do not. For the scalp examination in particular, then, you might ask your spouse or a friend to assist you.

Step 9

Sit down and prop one leg up on a chair or stool in front of you as shown. Using the hand-held mirror, examine the inside of the propped-up leg, beginning at the groin area and moving down the leg to your foot. Repeat the procedure for you other leg.

Step 10

Still sitting, cross one leg over the other. Use the hand-held mirror to examine the top of your foot, the toes, toenails, and spaces between the toes. Then look at the sole or bottom of your foot. Repeat the procedure for the other foot.

2. Practice recording the descriptions of various common skin lesions on your own arms and legs (freckles, warts, moles, and sores) by examining the color, size, configuration, and shape of any lesion you find.

3. Find an elderly client or friend or relative who will let you examine his or her skin, hair, and nails. Report your findings as they compare with those of a younger person's skin, hair, and nails.

INTERVIEWING AND RECORDING ASSESSMENT FINDINGS

Use the following Nursing History Checklist as your guide to interviewing and recording your findings in skin, hair, and nail assessment.

NURSING HISTORY CHECKLIST

Questions	Satisfactory data	Needs additional data	Data missing
Current Symptoms			
1. Skin problems (rashes, lesions, dryness, oiliness, drainage, bruising, swelling, pigmentation)			
2. Changes in lesion appearance			
3. Feeling changes (pain, pressure, itch, tingling)			
4. Hair loss or changes			
5. Nail changes			
6. Body odor problems			
Past History			
1. Previous problems with skin, hair, or nails (treatment and surgery)			
2. Allergic reactions			
Family History			
1. Family history of skin problems or skin cancer			
Lifestyle and Health Practices			
1. Exposure to sun or chemicals			
2. Daily care of skin, hair, and nails			
3. Usual diet and exercise patterns			

PERFORMING PHYSICAL ASSESSMENT

Use the following Physical Assessment Checklist as your guide to performing skin, hair, and nail assessment.

PHYSICAL ASSESSMENT CHECKLIST

Assessment Skill	Findings (Normal or Abnormal) and Notes		Performance (Satisfactory, Needs Improvement, Unsatisfactory)		
	N	A	S	N	U
1. Gather equipment (gloves, exam light, penlight, magnifying glass, centimeter ruler, Wood's lamp if available).	☐	☐	☐	☐	☐
2. Explain procedure to client.	☐	☐	☐	☐	☐
3. Ask client to gown.	☐	☐	☐	☐	☐

(continues)

PHYSICAL ASSESSMENT CHECKLIST *(Continued)*

Assessment Skill	Findings (Normal or Abnormal) and Notes		Performance (Satisfactory, Needs Improvement, Unsatisfactory)		
	N	**A**	**S**	**N**	**U**
Skin					
1. Note any distinctive odor.	☐	☐	☐	☐	☐
2. Inspect for generalized color variations (brownness, yellow, redness, pallor, cyanosis, jaundice, erythema, vitiligo)	☐	☐	☐	☐	☐
3. Inspect for skin breakdown (use staging criteria given in Chapter 9)	☐	☐	☐	☐	☐
4. Inspect for primary, secondary, or vascular lesions. (Note size, shape, location, distribution, and configuration.) Use Wood's lamp if fungus is suspected.	☐	☐	☐	☐	☐
5. Palpate lesions	☐	☐	☐	☐	☐
6. Palpate texture (rough, smooth) of skin, using palmar surface of three middle fingers.	☐	☐	☐	☐	☐
7. Palpate temperature (cool, warm, hot) and moisture (dry, sweaty, oily) of skin, using dorsal side of hand.	☐	☐	☐	☐	☐
8. Palpate thickness of skin with fingerpads.	☐	☐	☐	☐	☐
9. Palpate mobility and turgor by pinching up skin over sternum.	☐	☐	☐	☐	☐
10. Palpate for edema, pressing thumbs over feet or ankles.	☐	☐	☐	☐	☐
Scalp and Hair					
1. Inspect color.	☐	☐	☐	☐	☐
2. Inspect amount and distribution.	☐	☐	☐	☐	☐
3. Inspect and palpate for thickness, texture, oiliness, lesions, and parasites.	☐	☐	☐	☐	☐
Nails					
1. Inspect for grooming and cleanliness.	☐	☐	☐	☐	☐
2. Inspect for color and markings.	☐	☐	☐	☐	☐
3. Inspect shape.	☐	☐	☐	☐	☐
4. Palpate texture and consistency.	☐	☐	☐	☐	☐
5. Test for capillary refill.	☐	☐	☐	☐	☐
Analysis of Data					
1. Formulate nursing diagnoses (wellness, risk, actual).	☐	☐	☐	☐	☐
2. Formulate collaborative problems.	☐	☐	☐	☐	☐
3. Make necessary referrals.	☐	☐	☐	☐	☐

■ Chapter Post-test

MULTIPLE CHOICE

Choose the one best answer for each of the following multiple-choice questions.

_____ 1. An adult female client visits the clinic for the first time. The client has many bruises around her neck and face, and she tells the nurse that the bruises are the "result of an accident." The nurse suspects that the client may be experiencing

A. leukemia.

B. diabetes mellitus.

C. melanoma.

D. domestic abuse.

_____ 2. An adult male client visits the outpatient center and tells the nurse that he has been experiencing patchy hair loss. The nurse should further assess the client for

A. symptoms of stress.

B. recent radiation therapy.

C. pigmentation irregularities.

D. allergies to certain foods.

_____ 3. The nurse is instructing a group of high school students about risk factors associated with various skin cancers. The nurse should instruct the group that

A. melanoma skin cancers are the most common type of cancers.

B. African Americans are the least susceptible to skin cancers.

C. usually there are precursor lesions for basal cell carcinomas.

D. squamous cell carcinomas are most common on body sites with heavy sun exposure.

_____ 4. Squamous cell carcinoma is associated with

A. overall amount of sun exposure.

B. intermittent exposure to ultraviolet rays.

C. precursor lesions.

D. an increase in the rates of melanoma.

_____ 5. The nurse is assessing an African-American client's skin. After the assessment, the nurse should instruct the client that African-American persons are more susceptible to

A. skin cancers than persons of European origin.

B. melanomas if they reside in areas without ozone depletion.

C. chronic discoid lupus erythematosus.

D. genetic predisposition to melanomas.

_____ 6. A 20-year-old client visits the outpatient center and tells the nurse that he has been experiencing sudden generalized hair loss. After determining that the client has not received radiation or chemotherapy, the nurse should further assess the client for signs and symptoms of

A. hypothyroidism.

B. hyperthyroidism.

C. infectious conditions.

D. hypoparathyroidism.

_____ 7. A client visits the clinic for a routine physical examination. The nurse prepares to assess the client's skin. The nurse asks the client if there is a family history of skin cancer and should explain to the client that there is a genetic component with skin cancer, especially

A. basal cell carcinoma.

B. actinic keratoses.

C. squamous cell carcinoma.

D. malignant melanoma.

_____ 8. A female client visits the clinic and complains to the nurse that her skin feels "dry." The nurse should instruct the client that skin elasticity is related to adequate

A. calcium.

B. vitamin D.

C. carbohydrates.

D. fluid intake.

_____ 9. An adult white client visits the clinic for the first time. During assessment of the client's skin, the nurse should assess for central cyanosis by observing the client's

A. nailbeds.

B. oral mucosa.

C. sclera.

D. palms.

_____ 10. To assess for anemia in a dark-skinned client, the nurse should observe the client's skin for a color that appears

A. greenish.

B. ashen.

C. bluish.

D. olive.

_____ 11. The nurse is assessing a dark-skinned client who has been transported to the emergency room by ambulance. When the nurse observes that the client's skin appears pale, with blue-tinged lips and oral mucosa, the nurse should document the presence of

A. a great degree of cyanosis.

B. a mild degree of cyanosis.

C. lupus erythematosus.

D. hyperthyroidism.

_____ 12. A dark-skinned client visits the clinic because he "hasn't been feeling well." To assess the client's skin for jaundice, the nurse should inspect the client's

    A. abdomen.

    B. arms.

    C. legs.

    D. sclera.

_____ 13. While assessing the skin of an older adult client, the nurse observes that the client has small yellowish brown patches on her hands. The nurse should instruct the client that these spots are

    A. signs of an infectious process.

    B. caused by aging of the skin in older adults.

    C. precancerous lesions.

    D. signs of dermatitis.

_____ 14. While assessing an adult client's feet for fungal disease using a Wood's light, the nurse documents the presence of a fungus when the fluorescence is

    A. blue.

    B. red.

    C. yellow.

    D. purple.

_____ 15. The nurse assesses an older adult bedridden client in her home. While assessing the client's buttocks, the nurse observes that a small area of the skin is broken and resembles an erosion. The nurse should document the client's pressure ulcer as

    A. Stage I.

    B. Stage II.

    C. Stage III.

    D. Stage IV.

_____ 16. To assess an adult client's skin turgor, the nurse should

    A. press down on the skin of the feet.

    B. use the dorsal surfaces of the hands on the client's arms.

    C. use the fingerpads to palpate the skin at the sternum.

    D. use two fingers to pinch the skin under the clavicle.

_____ 17. While assessing the nails of an adult client, the nurse observes Beau's lines. The nurse should ask the client if he has had

    A. chemotherapy.

    B. radiation.

    C. a recent illness.

    D. steroid therapy.

_____ 18. While assessing the nails of an older adult, the nurse observes early clubbing. The nurse should further evaluate the client for signs and symptoms of

A. hypoxia.

B. trauma.

C. anemia.

D. infection.

_____ 19. While assessing an adult client, the nurse observes freckles on the client's face. The nurse should document the presence of

A. macules.

B. papules.

C. plaques.

D. bulla.

_____ 20. While assessing an adult client, the nurse observes an elevated, palpable, solid mass with a circumscribed border that measures 1 centimeter. The nurse documents this as a

A. plaque.

B. macule.

C. papule.

D. patch.

_____ 21. The nurse is preparing to examine the skin of an adult client with a diagnosis of herpes simplex. The nurse plans to measure the client's symptomatic lesions and measure the size of the client's

A. nodules.

B. bullae.

C. vesicles.

D. wheals.

_____ 22. An adult male client visits the clinic and tells the nurse that he thinks he has athlete's foot. The nurse observes that the client has linear cracks in the skin on both feet. The nurse should document the presence of

A. ulcers.

B. erosion.

C. scales.

D. fissures.

_____ 23. An African-American female client visits the clinic. She tells the nurse that she had her ears pierced several weeks ago, and an elevated, irregular, reddened mass has now developed at the earlobe. The nurse should document a

A. cyst.

B. lichenification.

C. bulla.

D. keloid.

_____ 24. A client who is an active outdoor swimmer recently received a diagnosis of discoid systemic lupus erythematosus. The client visits the clinic for a routine examination and tells the nurse that she continues to swim in the sunlight three times per week. She has accepted her patchy hair loss and wears a wig on occasion. A priority nursing diagnosis for the client is

A. ineffective individual coping related to changes in appearance.

B. anxiety related to loss of outdoor activities and altered skin appearance.

C. dry, flaking skin and dull, dry hair as a result of disease.

D. risk for ineffective health maintenance related to deficient knowledge of effects of sunlight on skin lesions.

CROSSWORD PUZZLE

Complete the following crossword puzzle to become more familiar with the terminology used with assessment of the skin, hair, and nails.

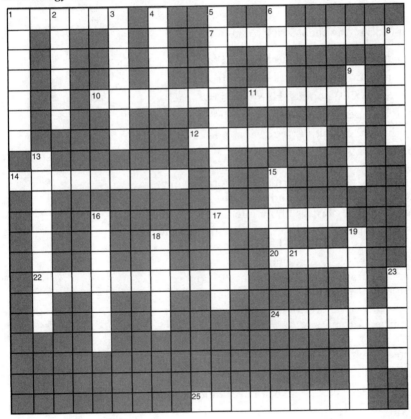

ACROSS

1. Solid, elevated, circumscribed, superficial lesion; 1 cm or less in diameter

7. Hardening of the skin, usually caused by edema

10. Linear crack in the skin

11. Flat, circumscribed lesion of the skin or mucous membrane; 1 cm or less in diameter

12. Spread out, widely dispersed

14. Swelling, discoloration and pain without a break in the skin; a bruise

17. Describes a lesion that forms a ring around a clear center of normal skin

20. Solid skin elevation extending into the dermal layer, more than 1 cm in diameter

22. Scratch or abrasion on the skin surface

24. Fluid-filled, elevated, superficial lesion, 1 cm or less in diameter

25. Tiny, flat, purple or red spots on the surface of the skin resulting from minute hemorrhage

DOWN CLUES

1. Vesicle or bulla that contains pus
2. Solid, elevated, circumscribed superficial lesion, more than 1 cm in diameter
3. Wearing away or destruction of the mucosal or epidermal surface; often develops into an ulcer
4. Congenital, pigmented area on the skin, e.g., mole, birthmark
5. Thickening of the skin characterized by accentuated skin markings
6. An elevated, circumscribed, fluid-filled lesion greater than 1 cm in diameter
8. Solid skin elevation that extends into the dermal layer, 1 cm or less in diameter

9. Hypertrophic scar tissue; prevalent in non-Caucasian races
13. Describes lesions that run together
15. Dried serum, blood, or purulent exudate on the skin
16. Decrease in size, or wasting
18. Small, thin flakes of epithelial cells
19. Hives; pruritic wheals, often transient and allergic in origin
21. Circumscribed crater on the surface of the skin or mucous membrane that leaves a wound
23. Elevated, solid, transient lesion; often irregularly shaped; an edematous response

CRITICAL THINKING AND CASE STUDIES

1. Discuss how you would assess for pallor, cyanosis, jaundice, and erythema in a dark-skinned client.

2. Read the following case study. Then analyze the client's risk for skin cancer.

   Mike McDaniel is a 47-year-old construction worker who has lived for 20 years in southern Florida. He has blond hair and tanned, leathery, freckled skin. He is 5 feet 10 inches tall and weighs 200 pounds. He smokes two packs of cigarettes and drinks a six-pack of beer per day. He describes himself as a "meat and potatoes man." He has a history of mild hypertension, and several members of his family have heart disease.

3. On the basis of the following case study assessment information, work through the steps of analyzing the data. Identify abnormal data and strengths in **subjective and objective findings**, assemble **cue clusters**, draw **inferences**, make possible **nursing diagnoses**, identify **defining characteristics, confirm or rule out** the diagnoses, and **document** your conclusions. Use the blank diagnostic analysis charts provided at the end of this book to guide your thinking. You may want to write on the chart or use separate paper. In either case, propose nursing diagnoses that are specific to the client in the case study. Identify collaborative problems, if any, for this client. Finally, identify data, if any, that point toward a medical problem requiring a referral.

   Evelyn Vaughn is a 47-year-old white woman who comes to the clinic for evaluation. She is a single mother and sells cosmetics in her home. She is lethargic and walks slowly into the room. She asks if she can have some "special lotion" for her dry skin.

   When interviewed, Evelyn states that her skin has been dry and scaly for the past several months, unrelieved by numerous moisturizers. She expresses concern about "fly-away hair that I can't do anything with" and about brittle, easily broken fingernails. When asked about medications, she explains that she is supposed to take Synthroid daily for "my low thyroid" but can't afford to get the prescription filled. She has a poor appetite, and with "not enough money to go around," she has been nibbling on crackers, lunch meat, and sodas daily. Exercise is out of the question because she lacks energy, and she is rarely able to get through a day without one or two 30-minute naps. Evelyn takes a shower and washes her hair using Ivory Soap and baby shampoo. She applies moisturizer to her skin and conditioner to her hair, but states that neither helps for any length of time. She keeps her nails cut short because they break so easily. She states that she has cut down on her cosmetic sales appointments because "I look like I never use my own products."

Your physical assessment reveals dry, flaking, skin that is cool to the touch and yellow tinged. Facial and periorbital edema are present. The client's facial expression is blank. She has multiple bruises on both forearms and anterior lower legs, which are in various stages of healing and tender when touched. Her scalp hair is dry and dull, and breaks easily. Her scalp is scaling. Sparse hair is noted in the axillae and the pubic area. Her fingernails are short and dry; her cuticles are dry and torn. Her toenails are thick and yellow.

■ Self-Reflection and Evaluation of Learner Objectives

After you have read Chapter 9 and completed the above quizzes and activities, please identify to what degree you have met each of the following chapter learning objectives. For those objectives that you have met partially or not at all, you will want to review chapter content for that learning objective.

Objective	Very much	Somewhat	Not at all
1. Describe the structures and functions of the skin.			
2. Discuss risk factors for skin cancer and ways to reduce these risk factors.			
3. Discuss the incidence of skin cancer across the cultures.			
4. Obtain an accurate nursing history of the client's skin, hair, and nails.			
5. Explain how to prepare the client and the equipment necessary to perform a skin, hair, and nail assessment.			
6. Describe the two physical examination techniques used to assess the skin.			
7. Assess the skin for color, breakdown, lesions, moisture, turgor, and edema.			
8. Describe the two physical examination techniques used to assess the hair and nails.			
9. Assess the scalp and hair for color, amount, distribution, condition, and texture.			
10. Assess the nails for grooming, color, markings, shape, texture, consistency, and capillary refill.			
11. Describe differences in hair color and texture that may be seen in ethnic groups.			
12. Describe changes that are common with aging of the skin, hair, and nails.			

For additional information on this book, be sure to visit *http://connection.lww.com.*

CHAPTER 10

Head and Neck Assessment

CHAPTER OVERVIEW

Assessment of the head and neck focuses on the cranium, face, thyroid gland, and lymph node structures contained within the head and neck. The client's health history is particularly important in this assessment because it provides clues to abnormalities that cannot be directly observed, for example, headaches and possible systemic problems . Use the following quizzes and activities to improve your head and neck assessment skills.

■ Chapter Pretest

MATCHING

Match the terms in the left column with the correct descriptions in the right column.

Term	Description
_____ 1. Parotid gland	A. The air passage extending from the throat and larynx to the main bronchi
_____ 2. Sublingual gland	B. Ringlike cartilage forming the lower and back part of the larynx
_____ 3. Trachea	C. Spinal accessory-contraction of trapezius and sternocleidomastoid muscles
_____ 4. Hyoid bone	
_____ 5. Cricoid cartilage	D. The largest of the three main parts of salivary glands, located on either side of the face, just below and in front of the ears
_____ 6. Thyroid gland	E. Paired muscles that allow movement and provide support to the head and neck
_____ 7. Cranial nerve XI	F. The largest of the endocrine glands, situated in the front and sides of the neck just below the thyroid cartilage
_____ 8. Trapezius and sternocleidomastoid	G. Cervical vertebra (C7) that can be easily palpated when the neck is flexed
_____ 9. Adam's apple	H. A salivary gland on either side of the tongue
_____10. Vertebra prominens	I. A horseshoe-shaped bone at the base of the tongue; the only bone in the body not directly attached to another bone
	J. The thyroid cartilage located just above the cricoid cartilage

LABELING ACTIVITY

Label the structures of the neck in the following figure.

Structures of the neck.

Label the structure indicated by the line; then match your answer with the label on the matching figure in chapter 10 of your textbook.

Label the neck muscles and landmarks in the following figure.

Neck muscles and landmarks.

Label the structure indicated by the line; then match your answer with the label on the matching figure in chapter 10 of your textbook.

Label the lymph nodes in the neck in the following figure.

Lymph nodes in the neck.

Label the structure indicated by the line; then match your answer with the label on the matching figure in chapter 10 of your textbook.

▪ Learner Activities

WORKING WITH PEERS IN LEARNING LAB

1. Refer in the textbook to Table 10-1, Kinds and Characteristics of Headaches. Interview your lab partner to determine whether he or she has ever had a headache. Determine the type it might have been, based on the information in Table 10-1.

2. Practice the correct method for palpating the thyroid gland on your lab partner. Discuss your findings: size, texture, smoothness, presence of nodules or masses.

3. Auscultate your lab partner's thyroid gland and carotid arteries. Discuss the significance of this exam and what would indicate an abnormality.

4. Demonstrate on your lab partner how to inspect and palpate the C7 vertebra. Discuss the changes that may occur with aging, such as kyphosis of the spine or dowager's hump.

5. Assess the lymph nodes of your lab partner. Discuss the normal and abnormal characteristics of the lymph nodes.

INTERVIEWING AND RECORDING ASSESSMENT FINDINGS

Use the following Nursing History Checklist as your guide to interviewing and recording your findings in a head and neck assessment.

NURSING HISTORY CHECKLIST

Questions	Satisfactory data	Needs additional data	Data missing
Current Symptoms			
1. Lumps or lesions on head or neck that do not heal or disappear			
2. Difficulty moving head or neck			
3. Facial or neck pain or frequent headaches			
4. Dizziness, lightheadedness, spinning sensation, or loss of consciousness			
Past History			
1. Previous head or neck problems/trauma/injury (surgery, medication, physical or radiation therapy); results			
Family History			
1. Family history of head and/or neck cancer			
2. Family history of migraine headaches			
Lifestyle and Health Practices			
1. Do you smoke or chew tobacco? Amount? Secondhand smoke?			
2. Do you wear a helmet or hard hat?			
3. Typical posture when relaxing, during sleep, and when working			
4. Type of recreational activities			
5. Satisfaction with appearance			

PERFORMING PHYSICAL ASSESSMENT

Use the following Physical Assessment Checklist as your guide to performing a
head and neck physical assessment.

PHYSICAL ASSESSMENT CHECKLIST

Assessment Skill	Findings (Normal or Abnormal) and Notes		Performance (Satisfactory, Needs Improvement, Unsatisfactory)		
	N	A	S	N	U
1. Gather equipment (gloves, penlight or flashlight, small glass of water, stethoscope).	☐	☐	☐	☐	☐
2. Explain procedure to client.	☐	☐	☐	☐	☐

Head and Face

1. Inspect head for size, shape, and configuration.	☐	☐	☐	☐	☐
2. Palpate head for consistency while wearing gloves.	☐	☐	☐	☐	☐
3. Inspect face for symmetry, features, movement, expression, and skin condition.	☐	☐	☐	☐	☐
4. Palpate temporal artery for tenderness and elasticity.	☐	☐	☐	☐	☐
5. Palpate temporomandibular joint for range of motion, swelling, tenderness, or crepitation by placing index finger over the front of each ear and asking client to open mouth. Ask if client has history of frequent headaches.	☐	☐	☐	☐	☐

Neck

1. Inspect neck while it is in a slightly extended position (and using a light) for position, symmetry, and presence of lumps and masses.	☐	☐	☐	☐	☐
2. Inspect movement of thyroid and cricoid cartilage and thyroid gland by having client swallow a small sip of water.	☐	☐	☐	☐	☐
3. Inspect cervical vertebrae by having client flex neck.	☐	☐	☐	☐	☐
4. Inspect neck range of motion by having client turn chin to right and left shoulder, touch each ear to the shoulder, touch chin to chest, and lift chin to ceiling.	☐	☐	☐	☐	☐
5. Palpate trachea by placing your finger in the sternal notch, feeling to each side, and palpating the tracheal rings.	☐	☐	☐	☐	☐
6. Palpate the thyroid gland.	☐	☐	☐	☐	☐
7. Auscultate thyroid gland for bruits if the gland is enlarged (use bell of stethoscope).	☐	☐	☐	☐	☐
8. Palpate lymph nodes for size/shape, delimitation, mobility, consistency, and tenderness (refer to display on characteristics of lymph nodes).	☐	☐	☐	☐	☐
a. Preauricular nodes (front of ears)	☐	☐	☐	☐	☐
b. Postauricular nodes (behind the ears)	☐	☐	☐	☐	☐
c. Occipital nodes (posterior base of skull)	☐	☐	☐	☐	☐
d. Tonsillar nodes (angle of the mandible, on the anterior edge of the sternocleidomastoid muscle)	☐	☐	☐	☐	☐

PHYSICAL ASSESSMENT CHECKLIST

Assessment Skill	Findings (Normal or Abnormal) and Notes		Performance (Satisfactory, Needs Improvement, Unsatisfactory)		
	N	**A**	**S**	**N**	**U**
e. Submandibular nodes (medial border of the mandible); don't confuse with the lobulated submandibular gland	☐	☐	☐	☐	☐
f. Submental nodes (a few centimeters behind the tip of the mandible); use one hand	☐	☐	☐	☐	☐
g. Superficial cervical nodes (superficial to the sternomastoid muscle)	☐	☐	☐	☐	☐
h. Posterior cervical nodes (posterior to the sternocleidomastoid and anterior to the trapezius in the posterior triangle)	☐	☐	☐	☐	☐
i. Deep cervical chain nodes (deep within and around the sternomastoid muscle)	☐	☐	☐	☐	☐
j. Supraclavicular nodes (hook fingers over clavicles and feel deeply between the clavicles and the sternomastoid muscles)	☐	☐	☐	☐	☐
Analysis of Data					
1. Formulate nursing diagnoses (wellness, risk, actual).	☐	☐	☐	☐	☐
2. Formulate collaborative problems.	☐	☐	☐	☐	☐
3. Make necessary referrals.	☐	☐	☐	☐	☐

■ Chapter Post-test

MULTIPLE CHOICE

_____ 1. The nurse assesses an adult client's head and neck. While examining the carotid arteries, the nurse assesses each artery individually in order to prevent a

A. reduction of the blood supply to the brain.

B. rapid rise in the client's pulse rate.

C. premature ventricular heart sound.

D. decreased pulse pressure.

_____ 2. A client visits the outpatient center with a complaint of sudden head and neck pain and stiffness. The client's oral temperature is 100 degrees F. The nurse suspects the client is experiencing symptoms of

A. migraine headache.

B. meningeal irritation.

C. trigeminal neuralgia.

D. otitis media.

_____ 3. While assessing the head and neck of an adult client, the client tells the nurse that she has been experiencing sharp, shooting facial pains that last from 10 to 20 seconds but are occurring more frequently. The nurse should refer the client for possible

   A. cancerous lesions.

   B. arterial occlusion.

   C. inner ear disease.

   D. trigeminal neuralgia.

_____ 4. A female client visits the clinic and tells the nurse that she frequently experiences severe, recurring headaches that sometimes last for several days and are accompanied by nausea and vomiting. The nurse determines that the type of headache the client is describing is a

   A. migraine headache.

   B. cluster headache.

   C. tension headache.

   D. tumor-related headache.

_____ 5. An adult client visits the clinic and tells the nurse that she has headaches recently that are intense and stabbing and often occur in the late evening. The nurse should document the presence of

   A. cluster headaches.

   B. migraine headaches.

   C. tension headaches.

   D. tumor-related headaches.

_____ 6. A client visits the clinic and tells the nurse that he is depressed because of a recent job loss. He complains of dull, aching, tight, and diffuse headaches that have lasted for several days. The nurse should document the client's

   A. cluster headaches.

   B. tumor-related headaches.

   C. migraine headaches.

   D. tension headaches.

_____ 7. An older client visits the clinic accompanied by his daughter. The daughter tells the nurse that her father has been experiencing severe headaches that usually begin in the morning and become worse when he coughs. The client tells the nurse that he feels dizzy when he has the headaches. The nurse refers the client for further evaluation because these symptoms are characteristic of a

   A. migraine headache.

   B. cluster headache.

   C. tension headache.

   D. tumor-related headache.

_____ 8. The nurse is preparing to perform a head and neck assessment of an adult client who has immigrated to the United States from Cambodia. The nurse should first

A. explain to the client why the assessment is necessary.

B. ask the client if touching the head is permissible.

C. determine if the client desires a family member present.

D. examine the lymph nodes of the neck before examining the head.

_____ 9. While assessing an adult client's skull, the nurse observes that the client's skull and facial bones are larger and thicker than usual. The nurse should assess the client for

A. parotid gland enlargement.

B. acromegaly.

C. Paget's disease.

D. Cushing's syndrome.

_____ 10. While assessing an adult client's skull, the nurse observes that the client's skull bones are acorn shaped and enlarged. The nurse should refer the client to a physician for possible

A. Cushing's syndrome.

B. scleroderma.

C. Paget's disease.

D. Parkinson's disease.

_____ 11. While assessing an adult client's head and neck, the nurse observes asymmetry in front of the client's earlobes. The nurse refers the client to the physician because the nurse suspects the client is most likely experiencing a/an

A. enlarged thyroid.

B. lymph node abscess.

C. neurologic disorder.

D. parotid gland enlargement.

_____ 12. The nurse is preparing to assess the neck of an adult client. To inspect movement of the client's thyroid gland, the nurse should ask the client to

A. inhale deeply.

B. swallow a small sip of water.

C. cough deeply.

D. flex the neck to each side.

_____ 13. While assessing an older adult client's neck, the nurse observes that the client's trachea is pulled to the left side. The nurse should

A. ask the client to flex his neck to the left side.

B. observe whether the client has difficulty swallowing water.

C. refer the client to a physician for further evaluation.

D. palpate the cricoid cartilage for smoothness.

_____ 14. The nurse is planning to assess an adult client's thyroid gland. The nurse should plan to

  A. ask the client to raise the chin.

  B. approach the client posteriorly.

  C. turn the client's neck slightly backward.

  D. place the fingers above the cricoid cartilage.

_____ 15. The nurse is preparing to assess the lymph nodes of an adult client. The nurse should instruct the client to

  A. lie in a supine position.

  B. lie in a side-lying position.

  C. stand upright in front of the nurse.

  D. sit in an upright position.

_____ 16. A female client visits the clinic and tells the nurse that she wants to "stay healthy." The nurse observes that the client has diffuse neck enlargement, is perspiring, and is quite fidgety. The client tells the nurse that she is "hungry all the time, but I have lost weight." A priority nursing diagnosis for the client is

  A. imbalanced nutrition: less than body requirements related to energy level.

  B. ineffective health maintenance related to increased metabolism and hunger.

  C. health-seeking behaviors related to verbalization of wanting to stay healthy.

  D. thyroid dysfunction related to neck swelling, perspiration, and fidgeting.

CRITICAL THINKING AND CASE STUDIES

1. Explain how head sizes and shapes vary among different cultures.

2. Ask students to discuss the significance of abnormal facial features described as asymmetric, moon-shaped, mask-like, tightened-hard, sunken, or pale and edematous.

3. Read the following case study:

   Marie Lawsome is a 26-year-old woman who is having frequent headaches in the frontal region of her head. She states that the headaches are dull and aching and have lasted days and occasionally weeks at a time. Ms. Lawsome reports using a warm cloth on her forehead and taking over-the-counter analgesics to help the pain, though the headaches are not always completely relieved.

   a. Describe the type of headache the client is most likely experiencing.

   b. Analyze what type of precipitating factors are likely to be revealed from your interview with Ms. Lawsome.

4. Based on the following case study assessment information, work through the steps of analyzing the data. Identify abnormal data and strengths in **subjective and objective findings**, assemble **cue clusters**, draw **inferences**, make possible

nursing diagnoses, identify **defining characteristics, confirm or rule out** the diagnoses, and **document** your conclusions. Use the blank diagnostic analysis charts provided at the end of this book to guide your thinking. You may want to write on the chart or use separate paper. In either case, propose nursing diagnoses that are specific to the client in the case study. Identify collaborative problems, if any, for this client. Finally, identify data, if any, that point toward a medical problem requiring a referral.

Dorothy Grant is a married, 38-year-old, white woman who has come to the office of the school nurse with what she describes as a migraine headache. She is employed by the school system as a music teacher for grades K through 8. She has had a long history of migraine headaches and experienced her first episode at the age of 16. Her father also had migraine headaches until his mid-50s. She is employed full time and is the mother of two school-aged children. She states that she is 5 feet 4 inches tall and weighs 140 pounds.

Dorothy relates that she has severe throbbing pain in the right temporal region. On a scale of 0 to 5 (with 5 being the worst), she rates her pain as a 4.5. She says she feels nauseated but denies vomiting. Although she is not currently experiencing visual disturbances, she did experience some about 2 hours ago. She describes them as beginning with a loss of her central field of vision, followed by flashing lights and then "orange and blue triangles moving from left to right" across her visual field. About an hour later, she experienced the pain. She also reports feeling "a little light-headed."

She took 600 mg of ibuprofen about 20 minutes ago. She states that sleeping for several hours is the best remedy. Although she usually sleeps well for seven hours a night, lately she has not been getting adequate sleep and has been "eating cheeseburgers on the run." This is a departure from her usual habit of eating three healthy meals a day with a snack of fruit or popcorn. Dorothy routinely attends a step aerobics class four to five times a week, although she has not attended any classes for the past 2 weeks because of late practices for the annual Christmas program. There is no other history of head or neck problems.

Physical assessment reveals that her skin is warm, pale, and dry to touch. Her voice trembles slightly when she is speaking. Her pulse is 78 beats/minute, her respirations are 24 breaths/minute, her blood pressure is 128/74 mm Hg, and her temperature is 98.8 degrees F. Her head and face are round and symmetric, with her head in a central position; no masses are noted. The client demonstrates normal range of motion of the head and neck, with no abnormal movements. The trachea is in the midline; the thyroid gland is nonpalpable. The cervical and supraclavicular lymph nodes are nonpalpable and nontender. The temporal area is tender to touch; the temporal artery is palpated. Test results of cranial nerves V, VII, and XI are normal. Her posture is erect, but she is holding her head with her hand.

■ Self-Reflection and Evaluation of Learner Objectives

After you have read Chapter 10 and completed the above quizzes and activities, please identify to what degree you have met each of the following chapter learning objectives. For those objectives that you have met partially or not at all, you will want to review chapter content for that learning objective.

Objective	Very much	Somewhat	Not at all
1. Describe the structures and functions of the head and neck.			
2. Obtain an accurate nursing history of the client's head and neck.			
3. Differentiate between the four major types of headaches.			
4. Obtain the necessary equipment, and prepare the client for an examination of the head and neck.			
5. Assess the head for size, shape, configuration, and consistency (hard and smooth).			
6. Assess the face for symmetry, features, movement, expression, and condition of the skin.			
7. Assess the temporal arteries for tenderness and elasticity.			
8. Describe age-related changes of the face and temporal arteries.			
9. Assess the temporomandibular joint for full range of motion, swelling, tenderness, and crepitation.			
10. Assess the neck for symmetry and range of motion.			
11. Assess the thyroid gland.			
12. Assess the trachea for position, and discuss its significance.			
13. Assess the lymph nodes in the head and neck for size, shape, delineation, mobility, consistency, and tenderness.			
14. Discuss various nursing diagnoses and collaborative problems commonly seen with assessment of the head and neck.			

For additional information on this book, be sure to visit *http://connection.lww.com.*

CHAPTER 11

Eye Assessment

CHAPTER OVERVIEW

Healthy eyes are essential for vision. Vision informs our lives, permits mobility, and assists learning. People without vision are handicapped indeed. This chapter reviews the structures and functions of the eye and the tests and techniques used by nurses to evaluate a client's visual acuity.

■ Chapter Pretest

MULTIPLE CHOICE

Choose the one best answer for each of the following multiple-choice questions.

_____ 1. The bony orbit and fat cushion of the eye serves as a
   A. caruncle.
   B. channel.
   C. protector.
   D. filter.

_____ 2. The tarsal plates of the upper eyelid contain
   A. meibomian glands.
   B. sebaceous glands.
   C. tear ducts.
   D. ocular muscles.

_____ 3. The conjunctiva of the eye is divided into the palpebral portion and the
   A. canthus portion.
   B. intraocular portion.
   C. nasolacrimal portion.
   D. bulbar portion.

_____ 4. Straight movements of the eye are controlled by the
   A. lacrimal muscles.
   B. oblique muscles.
   C. corneal muscles.
   D. rectus muscles.

_____ 5. The middle layer of the eye is known as the
   A. choroid layer.
   B. scleral layer.

C. retinal layer.

D. optic layer.

_____ 6. Photoreceptors of the eye are located in the eye's

A. ciliary body.

B. lens.

C. retina.

D. pupil.

_____ 7. The meibomian glands secrete

A. an oily substance to lubricate the eyes.

B. sweat.

C. hormones.

D. clear liquid tears.

_____ 8. The chambers of the eye contain aqueous humor, which helps to maintain intraocular pressure and

A. transmit light rays.

B. maintain the retinal vessels.

C. change refractory of the lens.

D. cleanse the cornea and the lens.

_____ 9. The optic nerves from each eyeball cross at the

A. optic chiasma.

B. vitreous humor.

C. optic disc.

D. visual cortex.

_____ 10. The functional reflex that allows the eyes to focus on near objects is termed

A. pupillary reflex.

B. accommodation.

C. refraction.

D. indirect reflex.

LABELING ACTIVITIES

Label the structures of the eye in the following figure.

Anatomy of the eye.

Label the structure indicated by the line; then match your answer with the label on the matching figure in chapter 11 of your textbook.

Label the structures of the eyelid in the following figure.

Eyelids

Label the structure indicated by the line; then match your answer with the label on the matching figure in chapter 11 of your textbook.

Label the structures of the lacrimal apparatus in the following figure.

Lacrimal apparatus.

Label the structure indicated by the line; then match your answer with the label on the matching figure in chapter 11 of your textbook

■ Learner Activities

After reading Chapter 11, participate in the following learning activities.

1. Read the Risk Factors display in Chapter 11 and determine your lab partner's risk for cataracts. Discuss ways to reduce these risks.

2. Prepare your lab partner for an eye exam (include positioning, explanation, and gathering of necessary equipment.

3. Interview your lab partner, using the questions in Chapter 11 under Collecting Subjective Data, Nursing History.

4. Obtain an ophthalmoscope and discuss how to use it, following the directions in Chapter 11.

5. Assess your lab partner's vision, using the Snellen chart. Interpret the results.

6. Assess your lab partner's visual fields. Describe your findings.

7. Inspect your lab partner's external eye structures. Describe the eyelids, lashes, position of eyeballs, bulbar conjunctiva and sclera, palpebral conjunctiva, and lacrimal apparatus.

8. Assess your lab partner's pupillary reaction to light and accommodation.

9. Use the ophthalmoscope to examine your lab partner's internal eye structures. Describe the red reflex, optic disc, retinal vessels, retinal background, fovea and macula, and anterior chamber.

INTERVIEWING AND RECORDING ASSESSMENT FINDINGS

Use the following Nursing History Checklist as your guide to interviewing and recording your findings in a vision and eye assessment of a peer, friend, or family member.

NURSING HISTORY CHECKLIST

Questions	Satisfactory data	Needs additional data	Data missing
Current Symptoms			
1. Recent changes in vision?			
2. Spots or floaters in front of eyes?			
3. Blind spots, halos, or rings around lights?			
4. Trouble seeing at night?			
5. Double vision?			
6. Eye pain?			
7. Redness or swelling in eyes?			
8. Excessive watering or tearing or other discharge from eyes?			
Past History			
1. Previous eye or vision problems (medication, surgery, laser treatments, corrective lenses)?			
Family History			
1. Family history of eye problems or vision loss?			
Lifestyle and Health Practices			
1. Exposure to chemicals, fumes, smoke, dust, flying sparks, etc.?			
2. Use of safety glasses?			
3. Use of sunglasses?			
4. Medications? (corticosteroids, lovastatin, pyridostigmine, quinidine, risperadol, and rifampin may have ocular side effects)			
5. Has vision loss affected ability to work or care for self or others?			
6. Date of last eye examination?			
7. Have glasses or contacts? Are they worn regularly?			
8. Live or work around frequent or continuous loud noise?			
9. Use of ear protection from noise or while in water?			

PERFORMING PHYSICAL ASSESSMENT

Use the following Physical Assessment Checklist to examine the eye of a peer, friend, or family member.

PHYSICAL ASSESSMENT CHECKLIST

Assessment Skill	Findings (Normal or Abnormal) and Notes		Performance (Satisfactory, Needs Improvement, Unsatisfactory)		
	N	A	S	N	U
1. Gather equipment (Snellen chart, handheld Snellen chart or near vision screener, penlight, opaque card, and ophthalmoscope).	☐	☐	☐	☐	☐
2. Explain procedures to client.	☐	☐	☐	☐	☐
Perform Vision Tests					
1. Distant visual acuity (with Snellen chart, normal acuity is 20/20 with or without corrective lenses).	☐	☐	☐	☐	☐
2. Near visual acuity (with a handheld vision chart, normal acuity is 14/14 with or without corrective lenses).	☐	☐	☐	☐	☐
3. Visual fields (use procedure discussed in text to test peripheral vision).	☐	☐	☐	☐	☐
Perform Extraocular Muscle Function Tests					
1. Corneal light reflex (using a penlight to observe parallel alignment of light reflection on corneas).	☐	☐	☐	☐	☐
2. Cover test (using an opaque card to cover an eye to observe for eye movement).	☐	☐	☐	☐	☐
3. Positions test (observing for eye movement).	☐	☐	☐	☐	☐
External Eye Structures					
1. Inspect eyelids and lashes (width and position of palpebral fissures, ability to close eyelids, direction of eyelids in comparison with eyeballs, color, swelling, lesions, or discharge).	☐	☐	☐	☐	☐
2. Inspect positioning of eyeballs (alignment in sockets, protruding or sunken).	☐	☐	☐	☐	☐
3. Inspect bulbar conjunctiva and sclera (clarity, color, and texture).	☐	☐	☐	☐	☐
4. Inspect the palpebral conjunctive (eversion of upper eyelid is usually performed only with complaints of eye pain or sensation of something in eye).	☐	☐	☐	☐	☐
5. Inspect the lacrimal apparatus over the lacrimal glands (lateral aspect of upper eyelid) and the puncta (medial aspect of lower eyelid). Observe for swelling, redness, or drainage.	☐	☐	☐	☐	☐
6. Palpate the lacrimal apparatus, noting drainage from the puncta when palpating the nasolacrimal duct.	☐	☐	☐	☐	☐
7. Inspect the cornea and lens by shining a light to determine transparency.	☐	☐	☐	☐	☐
8. Inspect the iris and pupil for shape and color of the	☐	☐	☐	☐	☐

PHYSICAL ASSESSMENT CHECKLIST

Assessment Skill	Findings (Normal or Abnormal) and Notes		Performance (Satisfactory, Needs Improvement, Unsatisfactory)		
	N	A	S	N	U
iris and size and shape of the pupil.					
9. Test pupillary reaction to light (in a darkened room, have client focus on a distant object, shine a light obliquely into the pupil, and observe the pupil's reaction to light-normally, pupils constrict).	☐	☐	☐	☐	☐
10. Test accommodation of pupils by shifting gaze from far to near (normally, pupils constrict).	☐	☐	☐	☐	☐
Internal Eye Structure					
1. Inspect the red reflex by using an ophthalmoscope to shine the light beam toward the client's pupil (normally, a red reflex is easily seen and should appear round with regular borders).	☐	☐	☐	☐	☐
2. Inspect the optic disc by using the ophthalmoscope focused on the pupil and moving very close to the eye. Rotate the diopter setting until the retinal structures are in sharp focus (observe disc for shape, color, size, and physiologic cup).	☐	☐	☐	☐	☐
3. Inspect the retinal vessels using the above technique (observe vessels for numbers of sets, color, diameter, arteriovenous ratio, and arteriovenous crossings).	☐	☐	☐	☐	☐
4. Inspect retinal background for color and the presence of lesions.	☐	☐	☐	☐	☐
5. Inspect the fovea and macula for lesions.	☐	☐	☐	☐	☐
6. Inspect the anterior chamber for transparency.	☐	☐	☐	☐	☐
Analysis of Data					
1. Formulate nursing diagnoses (wellness, risk, actual).	☐	☐	☐	☐	☐
2. Formulate collaborative problems.	☐	☐	☐	☐	☐
3. Make necessary referrals.	☐	☐	☐	☐	☐

■ Chapter Post-test

MULTIPLE CHOICE

Choose the one best answer for each of the following multiple-choice questions.

_____ 1. While assessing the eyes of an adult client, the nurse uses a wisp of cotton to stimulate the client's

    A. eyelid reflexes.

    B. refractory mechanism.

    C. lacrimal reflexes.

    D. corneal reflexes.

_____ 2. An adult client visits the clinic and tells the nurse that she has had a sudden change in her vision. The nurse should explain to the client that sudden changes in vision are often associated with

A. diabetes.

B. the aging process.

C. hypertension.

D. head trauma.

_____ 3. An adult client tells the nurse that he has been experiencing gradual vision loss. The nurse should

A. ask about the client's diet.

B. determine whether there is a history of glaucoma.

C. check the client's blood pressure.

D. ask the client if he has any known allergies.

_____ 4. A 45-year-old client tells the nurse that he occasionally sees spots in front of his eyes. The nurse should

A. tell the client that these often occur with aging.

B. refer the client to an ophthalmologist.

C. re-examine the client in 2 weeks.

D. assess the client for signs of diabetes.

_____ 5. An adult client tells the nurse that her peripheral vision isn't what it used to be and she has a blind spot in her left eye. The nurse should refer the client for evaluation of possible

A. glaucoma.

B. increased intracranial pressure.

C. bacterial infection.

D. migraine headaches.

_____ 6. A client visits the local clinic after experiencing head trauma. The client tells the nurse that he has a consistent blind spot in his right eye. The nurse should

A. examine the area of head trauma.

B. refer the client to an ophthalmologist.

C. assess the client for double vision.

D. ask the client if he sees "halos."

_____ 7. A client tells the nurse that she has difficulty seeing while driving at night. The nurse should explain to the client that night blindness is often associated with

A. retinal deterioration.

B. head trauma.

C. migraine headaches.

D. vitamin A deficiency.

_____ 8. An adult client visits the clinic and tells the nurse that he has been experiencing double vision for the past few days. The nurse refers the client to a physician for evaluation of possible

A. glaucoma.

B. increased intracranial pressure.

C. hypertension.

D. ophthalmic migraine.

_____ 9. An adult client tells the nurse that she frequently experiences burning and itching of both eyes. The nurse should assess the client for

A. a foreign body.

B. recent trauma.

C. blind spots.

D. allergies.

_____ 10. An adult client visits the outpatient clinic and tells the nurse that he has a throbbing, aching pain in his right eye. The nurse should assess the client for

A. recent exposure to irritants.

B. increased intracranial pressure.

C. excessive tearing.

D. a foreign body in the eye.

_____ 11. An adult client visits the clinic and tells the nurse that he has had excessive tearing in his left eye. The nurse should assess the client's eye for

A. viral infection.

B. double vision.

C. allergic reactions.

D. lacrimal obstruction.

_____ 12. The nurse is caring for a healthy adult client with no history of vision problems in the past. The nurse should tell the client that a thorough eye examination is recommended every

A. year.

B. 2 years.

C. 3 years.

D. 4 years.

_____ 13. An adult client tells the nurse that his eyes are painful because he left his contact lenses in too long the day before yesterday. The nurse should instruct the client that prolonged wearing of contact lenses can lead to

A. retinal damage.

B. cataracts.

C. myopia.

D. corneal damage.

_____ 14. An adult client tells the nurse that his father had cataracts. He asks the nurse about risk factors for cataracts. The nurse should instruct the client that a potential risk factor is

A. lack of vitamin C in the diet.

B. ultraviolet light exposure.

C. obesity.

D. use of antibiotics.

_____ 15. The nurse is preparing to examine an adult client's eyes, using a Snellen chart. The nurse should

A. position the client 20 feet away from the chart.

B. ask the client to remove his glasses.

C. ask the client to read each line with both eyes open.

D. instruct the client to begin reading from the bottom of the chart.

_____ 16. A client has tested 20/40 on the distant visual acuity test using a Snellen chart. The nurse should

A. document the results in the client's record.

B. ask the client to read a handheld vision chart.

C. ask the client to return in 2 weeks for another examination.

D. refer the client to an optometrist.

_____ 17. The nurse has tested an adult client's visual fields and determined that the temporal field is 90 degrees in both eyes. The nurse should

A. refer the client for further evaluation.

B. examine the client for other signs of glaucoma.

C. ask the client if there is a genetic history of blindness.

D. document the findings in the client's records.

_____ 18. The nurse has tested the near visual acuity of a 45-year-old client. The nurse explains to the client that the client has impaired near vision and discusses a possible reason for the condition. The nurse determines that the client has understood the instructions when the client says that presbyopia is usually due to

A. congenital cataracts.

B. decreased accommodation.

C. muscle weakness.

D. constant misalignment of the eyes.

_____ 19. While assessing the eye of an adult client, the nurse observes an inward turning of the client's left eye. The nurse should document the client's

A. esotropia.

B. strabismus.

C. phoria.

D. exotropia.

_____ 20. The nurse is examining an adult client's eyes. The nurse has explained the positions test to the client. The nurse determines that the client needs further instructions when the client says that the positions test

A. assesses the muscle strength of the eye.

B. assesses the functioning of the cranial nerves innervating the eye muscles.

C. requires the covering of each eye separately.

D. requires the client to focus on an object.

CRITICAL THINKING AND CASE STUDIES

1. A 62-year-old woman arrives for an eye examination complaining of blurred vision. You find out from the nursing history that she has smoked a half pack of cigarettes a day for 30 years and spends a lot of time at the beach. She also tells you that she is taking medication for high blood pressure but often forgets to take it. Describe what areas you will focus on during her eye examination, and analyze her possible risk factors for eye disorders.

2. On the basis of the following case study assessment information, work through the steps of analyzing the data. Identify abnormal data and strengths in **subjective and objective findings**, assemble **cue clusters**, draw **inferences**, make possible **nursing diagnoses**, identify **defining characteristics, confirm or rule out** the diagnoses, and **document** your conclusions. Use the blank diagnostic analysis charts provided at the end of this book to guide your thinking. You may want to write on the chart or use separate paper. In either case, propose nursing diagnoses that are specific to the client in the case study. Identify collaborative problems, if any, for this client. Finally, identify data, if any, that point toward a medical problem requiring a referral.

Mrs. Hira is a 68-year-old woman of Indian descent who comes to the community outpatient clinic for evaluation because she states that she "can't see as well as I used to." She has been retired from the telephone company for 3 years. Her 71-year-old husband had a major stroke 1 year ago, and she is solely responsible for his care. They live in a small, one-story house and have a car, which Mrs. Hira uses for grocery shopping and to go to church. Their daughter and her family live 200 miles away.

When interviewed, Mrs. Hira reports progressive changes in her vision over the past 5 months. She reports changes in her vision as "blurring that seems to be getting worse" and reports a halo effect at night when looking at lights. She said that she doesn't drive much at night any more because of this. She has worn glasses for reading for the past 20 years. She denies eye pain, swelling, excessive tearing, or discharge. Mrs. Hira says that she had an eye examination 4 years ago. She states that she has never experienced any trauma to her eyes or head and has never had any serious eye problems or surgery. She doesn't know of any family history of eye problems.

Your physical assessment reveals distant visual acuity in the right eye (OD) 20/40, in the left eye (OS) 20/40. No lid lag is noted. The extraocular muscles are intact. The visual fields are equal to the examiner's. No excessive tearing or blinking is noted. The conjunctivae are smooth and without redness. The pupils are bilaterally round, equal in size, and reactive to light and accommodation. No nystagmus is noted. You are unable to assess the red reflex or perform an ophthalmic examination because of bilateral opacities of the lens.

■ Self-Reflection and Evaluation of Learner Objectives

After you have read Chapter 11 and completed the above quizzes and activities, please identify to what degree you have met each of the following chapter learning objectives. For those objectives that you have met partially or not at all, you will want to review chapter content for that learning objective.

Objective	Very much	Somewhat	Not at all
1. Describe the structures and function of the eye.			
2. Discuss the risk factors for cataracts and ways to reduce those risk factors.			
3. Describe the equipment and client preparation necessary for an eye exam.			
4. Demonstrate the proper method for testing a client's distal and near vision.			
5. Demonstrate the testing of visual fields.			
6. Demonstrate assessment of the client's extraocular muscle function.			
7. Demonstrate assessment of the client's external eye structures.			
8. Demonstrate examination of the client's pupillary reaction to light and accommodation.			
9. Use the ophthalmoscope to inspect the client's Red reflex Optic disc Retinal vessels Retinal background Fovea and macula Anterior chamber			

For additional information on this book, be sure to visit *http://connection.lww.com.*

CHAPTER 12

Ear Assessment

CHAPTER OVERVIEW

The sense organ of hearing and equilibrium is the ear, which has many parts, in particular the external ear, the middle ear, and the inner ear. Healthy ears are essential to effective communication and balance. This chapter reviews the structure and functions connected with hearing and balance as well as the techniques used in physical assessment of hearing acuity and sound conduction.

■ Chapter Pretest

MULTIPLE CHOICE

Choose one best answer for each of the following multiple choice questions.

_____ 1. The cone of light is located in the

    A. inner ear.

    B. middle ear.

    C. external ear.

    D. semicircular canal.

_____ 2. The ossicles contained in the middle ear include the malleus, the incus, and the

    A. pars tensa.

    B. pars flaccida.

    C. umbo.

    D. stapes

_____ 3. Sensory receptors in the ear that help to maintain both static and dynamic equilibrium are located in the semicircular canals and the

    A. vestibule.

    B. tympanic membrane.

    C. cone of light.

    D. eustachian tube.

_____ 4. In the hearing pathway, hair cells of the spiral organ of Corti are stimulated by movement of

    A. fluid.

    B. sound.

    C. air.

    D. bone.

_____ 5. The transmission of sound waves through the external ear and middle
       ear is known as
     A. perceptive hearing.
     B. conductive hearing.
     C. external hearing.
     D. connective hearing.

_____ 6. Transmission of sound waves in the inner ear is known as
     A. conducive hearing.
     B. tympanic hearing.
     C. neuromotor hearing.
     D. perceptive hearing.

LABELING ACTIVITY

Label the structures of the ear in the following figure.

External, middle, and inner ear.

Label the structure indicated by the line; then match your answer with the label on the matching figure in chapter 12 of your textbook.

Label the structures of the tympanic membrane in the following figure.

Right tympanic membrane.

Label the structure indicated by the line; then match your answer with the label on the matching figure in chapter 12 of your textbook.

Label the pathways of hearing in the following figure.

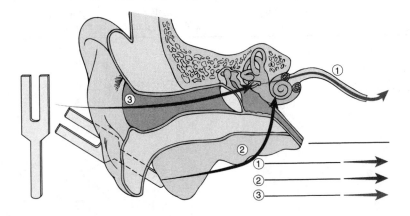

Pathways of hearing.

Label the structure indicated by the line; then match your answer with the label on the matching figure in chapter 12 of your textbook.

■ Learner Activities

WORKING WITH PEERS IN LEARNING LAB

After reading Chapter 12, participate in the following learning activities.

1. Obtain an otoscope. Read How to Use an Otoscope in Chapter 12 of your textbook. Practice handling and operating the otoscope before using it to inspect the eardrum of your lab partner. Report your findings.

2. Examine the ears of an elderly client, friend, or relative, and report your findings. Compare your findings with the variation of findings in the elderly discussed in the text.

3. Obtain a tuning fork. Practice using it after reading the instructions in your textbook. Explain how to perform both the Weber test and the Rinne test, and discuss the significance of each. Perform the Weber and Rinne tests on your lab partner, and report your findings.

INTERVIEWING AND RECORDING ASSESSMENT FINDINGS

Use the following Nursing History Checklist to interview a peer friend or family member regarding hearing and ear health.

NURSING HISTORY CHECKLIST

Questions	Satisfactory data	Needs additional data	Data missing
Current Symptoms			
1. Recent changes in hearing (if yes, were all or just some sounds affected)?			
2. Ear discharge (if yes, amount/odor)?			
3. Ear pain (if yes, is there accompanying sore throat, sinus infection, or problem with teeth or gums)?			
4. Ringing or crackling in ears?			

(continues)

NURSING HISTORY CHECKLIST (Continued)

Questions	Satisfactory data	Needs additional data	Data missing
Past History			
1. Previous ear or hearing problems such as infections, trauma, or earaches (medications, surgery, hearing aids)?			
Family History			
1. Family history of ear problems or hearing loss?			
Lifestyle and Health Practices			
1. Live or work around frequent or continuous loud noise?			
2. Use of ear protection from noise or while in water?			
3. Has hearing loss affected ability to work or care for self or others?			

PERFORMING PHYSICAL ASSESSMENT

Use the following Physical Assessment Checklist as your guide to performing a hearing and ear assessment for a peer, friend, or family member.

PHYSICAL ASSESSMENT CHECKLIST

Assessment Skill	Findings (Normal or Abnormal) and Notes		Performance (Satisfactory, Needs Improvement, Unsatisfactory)		
	N	A	S	N	U
External Ear Structures					
1. Inspect the auricle, tragus, and lobule for size and shape, position, lesions/discoloration, and discharge.	☐	☐	☐	☐	☐
2. Palpate the auricle and mastoid process for tenderness.	☐	☐	☐	☐	☐
Otoscopic Examination					
1. Inspect the external auditory canal with the otoscope for discharge, color and consistency of cerumen, color and consistency of canal walls, and nodules.	☐	☐	☐	☐	☐
2. Inspect the tympanic membrane, using the otoscope, for color and shape, consistency, and landmarks.	☐	☐	☐	☐	☐
3. Have client perform the Valsalva maneuver, and observe the center of the tympanic membrane for a flutter. (Do not do this procedure on the older client, as it may interfere with equilibrium and cause dizziness.)	☐	☐	☐	☐	☐

PHYSICAL ASSESSMENT CHECKLIST

Assessment Skill	Findings (Normal or Abnormal) and Notes		Performance (Satisfactory, Needs Improvement, Unsatisfactory)		
	N	A	S	N	U
Hearing and Equilibrium Tests					
1. Perform the whisper test by having the client place a finger on the tragus of one ear. Whisper a two-syllable word 1 to 2 feet behind the client. Repeat on the other ear.	☐	☐	☐	☐	☐
2. Perform the Weber test by using a tuning fork placed on the center of the head or forehead and asking whether the client hears the sound better in one ear or the same in both ears	☐	☐	☐	☐	☐
3. Perform the Rinne test by using a tuning fork and placing the base on the client's mastoid process. When the client no longer hears the sound, note the time interval, and move it in front of the external ear. When the client no longer hears a sound, note the time interval.	☐	☐	☐	☐	☐
4. Perform the Romberg test to evaluate equilibrium. With feet together and arms at the side, close eyes for 20 seconds. Observe for swaying. (Refer to text, chapters 12 and 22.)	☐	☐	☐	☐	☐
Analysis of Data					
1. Formulate nursing diagnoses (wellness, risk, actual).	☐	☐	☐	☐	☐
2. Formulate collaborative problems.	☐	☐	☐	☐	☐
3. Make necessary referrals.	☐	☐	☐	☐	☐

■ Chapter Post-test

MULTIPLE CHOICE

_____ 1. An adult client visits the clinic and complains of tinnitus. The nurse should ask the client if she has been

A. dizzy.

B. hypotensive.

C. taking antibiotics.

D. experiencing ear drainage.

_____ 2. An adult client tells the nurse that his 80-year-old father is almost completely deaf. After an explanation to the client about risk factors for hearing loss, the nurse determines that the client needs further instruction when the client says

A. "There is a genetic predisposition to hearing loss."

B. "Certain cultural groups have a higher rate of hearing loss."

C. "It is difficult to prevent hearing loss or worsening of hearing."

D. "Chronic otitis media has been associated with hearing loss."

_____ 3. The nurse is planning to perform an eye and ear examination on an adult client. After explaining the procedures to the client, the nurse should

    A. ask the client to remain standing.

    B. show the client the otoscope.

    C. ask the client to remove his contact lenses.

    D. observe the client's response to the explanations.

_____ 4. The nurse is preparing to examine the ears of an adult client with an otoscope. The nurse should plan to

    A. ask the client to tilt the head slightly forward.

    B. release the auricle during the examination.

    C. use a speculum that measures 10 mm in diameter.

    D. firmly pull the auricle out, up, and back.

_____ 5. While assessing the ears of an adult client, the nurse observes bloody drainage in the client's ear. The nurse should

    A. document the finding in the client's chart.

    B. determine whether a foreign body is present in the ear.

    C. assess the client for further signs of otitis media.

    D. refer the client to a physician.

_____ 6. While assessing the ears of an adult client, the nurse observes that the tympanic membrane is completely immobile. The nurse should further assess the client for signs and symptoms of

    A. infection.

    B. skull injury.

    C. vestibular disorders.

    D. healed perforations.

_____ 7. The nurse is planning to conduct the Weber test on an adult male client. To perform this test, the nurse should plan to

    A. strike a tuning fork and place it at the base of the client's mastoid process.

    B. whisper a word with two distinct syllables to the client.

    C. ask the client to close his eyes while standing with feet together.

    D. strike a tuning fork and place it on the center of the client's head or forehead.

_____ 8. The nurse has performed the Rinne test on an older adult client. After the test, the client reports that her bone conduction sound was heard longer than the air conduction sound. The nurse determines that the client is most likely experiencing

    A. normal hearing.

    B. sensorineural hearing loss.

    C. conductive hearing loss.

    D. central hearing loss.

MATCHING

Match the terms in the left column with the correct descriptions in the right column.

Term	Description
_____ 1. Conductive hearing	A. Gradual hearing loss
_____ 2. Perceptive or sensorineural hearing	B. Infection of the ear canal
	C. Drainage from the ear
_____ 3. Presbycusis	D. Ringing in the ears
_____ 4. Otorrhea	E. Earache
_____ 5. Otalgia	F. Ear wax
_____ 6. Tinnitus	G. Transmission of sound waves through the external and middle ear
_____ 7. Vertigo	H. True spinning motion
_____ 8. Swimmer's ear	I. Transmission of sound waves in the inner ear.
_____ 9. Cerumen	

CRITICAL THINKING AND CASE STUDIES

1. Discuss normal findings and what may be occurring if tenderness is present during the ear exam.

2. Discuss ethnic variations that may be found during the ear exam.

3. Discuss the differences between conductive and sensorineural hearing.

4. Explain the meaning of the findings identified during a Weber test and a Rinne test.

5. On the basis of the following case study assessment information, work through the steps of analyzing the data. Identify abnormal data and strengths in **subjective and objective findings**, assemble **cue clusters**, draw **inferences**, make possible **nursing diagnoses**, identify **defining characteristics, confirm or rule out** the diagnoses, and **document** your conclusions. Use the blank diagnostic analysis charts provided at the end of this book to guide your thinking. You may want to write on the chart or use separate paper. In either case, propose nursing diagnoses that are specific to the client in the case study. Identify collaborative problems, if any, for this client. Finally, identify data, if any, that point toward a medical problem requiring a referral.

Jack Jones, a 28-year-old man, currently works in an industrial plant as a supervisor. He noticed lately that he is having trouble hearing conversations with his friends, but of even more concern is that he misunderstands his workers when they are giving him information about the projects they are working on. He denies any major current or past illnesses—"just the kid stuff, you know, colds and fevers. I do have trouble with ringing in my ears." He admits that when he was in his teens he frequently attended music concerts that were often loud, and he still goes occasionally. He tells you that he likes to listen to loud— "the louder the better"—rock music, using tight earphones. When he watches TV in the evening, he has to turn up the volume to hear clearly.

■ Self-Reflection and Evaluation of Learner Objectives

After you have read Chapter 12 and completed the above quizzes and activities, please identify to what extent you have met each of the following chapter learning objectives. For those that you have met partially or not at all, you will want to review chapter content for that learning objective.

Objective	Very much	Somewhat	Not at all
1. Describe the functions and the structures of the ear.			
2. Describe the equipment necessary to perform an ear assessment.			
3. Assess the external ear structures by inspecting the auricle, tragus, and lobule and by palpating the auricle and mastoid process.			
4. Describe the expected changes with aging of the ear.			
5. Use the otoscope to inspect the auditory canal and the tympanic membrane.			
6. Perform three tests-the whisper, Weber, and Rinne tests-to assess the client's hearing.			
7. Perform the Romberg test to assess the client's equilibrium.			
8. Discuss various nursing diagnoses and collaborative problems related to assessment of the ears.			

For additional information on this book, be sure to visit *http://connection.lww.com.*

CHAPTER 13

Mouth, Nose, Throat, and Sinus Assessment

CHAPTER OVERVIEW

The mouth, nose, throat, and sinuses are the structures associated with eating, smell and taste, swallowing, speech, and purifying and warming the air that is transported to the lungs. Use the following activities and quizzes to review the structure and function of these very important tissues.

■ Chapter Pretest

MULTIPLE CHOICE

Choose the one best answer for each of the following multiple-choice questions.

_____ 1. The roof of the oral cavity of the mouth is formed by the anterior hard palate and the

    A. teeth.

    B. gums.

    C. muscles.

    D. soft palate.

_____ 2. An extension of the soft palate of the mouth, which hangs in the posterior midline of the oropharynx, is the

    A. uvula.

    B. frenulum.

    C. taste buds.

    D. sublingual fold.

_____ 3. The tongue is attached to the hyoid bone and styloid process of the temporal bone and is connected to the floor of the mouth by the

    A. mandible.

    B. frenulum.

    C. gums.

    D. soft palate.

_____ 4. The submandibular glands open under the tongue through openings called

    A. parasinal ducts.

    B. Stensen's ducts.

    C. Wharton's ducts.

    D. lacrimonasal ducts.

_____ 5. The rich blood supply of the nose serves to
   A. help propel moist air to the body.
   B. propel debris to the throat.
   C. filter large particles from the air.
   D. warm the inspired air.

LABELING ACTIVITIES

Label the following structures of the mouth.

Stuctures of the mouth.

Label the structure indicated by the line; then match your answer with the label on the matching figure in chapter 13 of your textbook.

Label the following teeth.

Teeth.

Label the structure indicated by the line; then match your answer with the label on the matching figure in chapter 13 of your textbook.

Label the structures of the salivary glands.

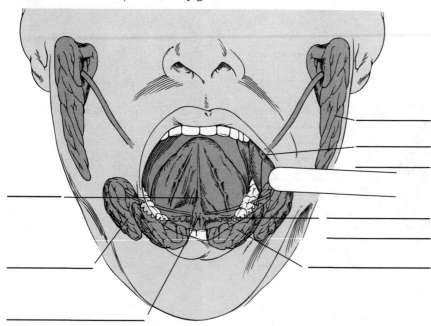

_____ Salivary glands.

Label the structure indicated by the line; then match your answer with the label on the matching figure in chapter 13 of your textbook.

Label the structures of the nasal cavity and throat.

Nasal cavity and throat.

Label the structure indicated by the line; then match your answer with the label on the matching figure in chapter 13 of your textbook.

Label the structures of the paranasal sinuses.

Paranasal sinuses.

Label the structure indicated by the line; then match your answer with the label on the matching figure in chapter 13 of your textbook.

■ Learner Activities

WORKING WITH PEERS IN LEARNING LAB

After reading Chapter 13, participate in the following learning activities.

1. Review the information in the Risk Factors display in Chapter 13. Determine your own risk for oral cancer. Next, discuss various behaviors—cultural and otherwise—that contribute to oral cancer.

2. Find an elderly client, friend, or relative whose mouth, nose, throat, and sinuses you can examine. Discuss with peers your findings as they compare with those of a younger person's mouth, nose, throat, and sinuses.

INTERVIEWING AND RECORDING ASSESSMENT FINDINGS

Use the following Nursing History Checklist to interview and record your findings from a mouth, nose, throat, nd sinus assessment of a peer, friend, or family member.

NURSING HISTORY CHECKLIST

Questions	Satisfactory data	Needs additional data	Data missing
Current Symptoms			
1. Mouth problems (tongue or mouth sores or lesions, gum or mouth redness, swelling, bleeding, or pain)?			
2. Sinus problems (pain over sinuses, postnasal drip)?			
3. Nose problems (nosebleeds, stuffy nose, cannot breath through one or both nostrils, change in ability to smell or taste)?			

(continues)

NURSING HISTORY CHECKLIST *(Continued)*

Questions	Satisfactory data	Needs additional data	Data missing
Past History			
1. Previous problems with mouth, nose, throat, or sinuses (surgeries or treatment; how much and how often)?			
2. Use of nasal sprays?			
3. History of tooth grinding?			
4. Last dental exam? Fit of dentures?			
Family History			
1. Family history of oral, nasal, or sinus cancer or chronic problems?			
Lifestyle and Health Practices			
1. Daily practice of oral care, tooth care, or denture care?			
2. Usual diet?			
3. History of smoking, use of, how much, and how often?			
4. Use of alcohol (how much and how often)?			

PERFORMING PHYSICAL ASSESSMENT

Use the following Physical Assessment Checklist to guide your mouth, nose, throat, and sinus examination of a peer, friend, or family member.

PHYSICAL ASSESSMENT CHECKLIST

Assessment Skill	Findings (Normal or Abnormal) and Notes		Performance (Satisfactory, Needs Improvement, Unsatisfactory)		
	N	A	S	N	U
1. Gather equipment (gloves, cotton gauze pads, penlight, speculum attached to otoscope, tongue blade).	☐	☐	☐	☐	☐
2. Explain procedure to client.	☐	☐	☐	☐	☐
Mouth					
1. Note any distinctive odors.	☐	☐	☐	☐	☐
2. Inspect and palpate lips, buccal mucosa, gums, and tongue for color variations (pallor, redness, white patches, bluish hue), moisture, tissue consistency, or lesions (induration, roughness, vesicles, crusts, plaques, nodules, ulcers, cracking, patches, bleeding, Koplik's spots, cancer sores), Stensen's and Wharton's ducts.	☐	☐	☐	☐	☐
3. Inspect gums for hyperplasia, blue-black line.	☐	☐	☐	☐	☐
4. Inspect teeth for number and shape, color (white, brown, yellow, chalky white areas), occlusion.	☐	☐	☐	☐	☐

PHYSICAL ASSESSMENT CHECKLIST

Assessment Skill	Findings (Normal or Abnormal) and Notes		Performance (Satisfactory, Needs Improvement, Unsatisfactory)		
	N	A	S	N	U
5. Inspect and palpate tongue for color, texture and consistency (black, hairy, white patches, smooth, reddish, shiny without papillae), moisture, and size (enlarged or very small).	☐	☐	☐	☐	☐
Throat					
1. Inspect the throat for color, consistency, torus palatinus, uvula (singular).	☐	☐	☐	☐	☐
2. Inspect the tonsils for color and consistency; grading scale (1+, 2+, 3+, 4+).	☐	☐	☐	☐	☐
Nose					
1. Inspect and palpate the external nose for color, shape, consistency, tenderness, and patency of airflow.	☐	☐	☐	☐	☐
2. Inspect the internal nose for color, swelling, exudate, bleeding, ulcers, perforated septum, or polyps.	☐	☐	☐	☐	☐
Sinuses					
1. Palpate the sinuses for tenderness.	☐	☐	☐	☐	☐
2. Percuss and transilluminate the sinuses for air versus fluid or pus.	☐	☐	☐	☐	☐
Analysis of Data					
1. Formulate nursing diagnoses (wellness, risk, actual).	☐	☐	☐	☐	☐
2. Formulate collaborative problems.	☐	☐	☐	☐	☐
3. Make necessary referrals.	☐	☐	☐	☐	☐

CRITICAL THINKING AND CASE STUDIES

1. Discuss how you would differentiate allergic conditions from infections.

2. Read the following case study. Analyze the client's risk factors for oral cancer.

   Clara Burton is a 25-year-old college student with chronic rhinitis. She says that she has a history of sinus infections about twice a year. She smokes two packs of cigarettes a day, drinks beer every weekend and occasionally during the week, and eats a poorly balanced diet on the run. Her father smoked a pipe and had lip cancer.

3. On the basis of the following case study assessment information, work through the steps of analyzing the data. Identify abnormal data and strengths in **subjective and objective findings**, assemble **cue clusters**, draw **inferences**, make possible **nursing diagnoses**, identify **defining characteristics**, **confirm or rule out** the diagnoses, and **document** your conclusions.
   Use the blank diagnostic analysis charts provided at the end of this book to guide your thinking. You may want to write on the chart or use separate paper. In either case, propose nursing diagnoses that are specific to the client in the

case study. Identify collaborative problems, if any, for this client. Finally, identify data, if any, that point toward a medical problem requiring a referral.

Alice Kennedy is a 50-year-old divorced woman with a medical diagnosis of carcinoma of the sphenoid sinus and nasal pharynx. She has been referred by the physician to the hospital's home health service for weekly skilled nursing visits by an R.N. She lives in her own home and is currently being cared for by her younger sister. Alice has two grown sons. One son lives close by; the other lives in another state.

Ms. Kennedy is currently being treated with radiation therapy, which she receives three times weekly. She states that she is experiencing some pain across the bridge of her nose (2 on a scale of 0 to 5, with 5 being the worst). She uses cold compresses to help relieve the pain. Three small oral ulcers approximately 3 to 5 centimeters wide are noted on the left buccal mucosa. Ms. Kennedy reports that she has no difficulty swallowing, but the sores are painful when she eats, especially when she eats citrus fruits. She uses a soft-bristled toothbrush and brushes her teeth gently after eating, and she tries to avoid irritating food. The findings in the rest of the oral examination are within normal limits.

The nasal examination reveals a slightly reddened color of the nose, with some tenderness noted across the bridge of the nose. There is no occlusion of either nostril. The nasal septum is intact, with no ulcers or perforations. The nasal mucosa is red and slightly swollen. Both frontal and maxillary sinuses transilluminate; the frontal sinus area is slightly tender to palpation.

Ms. Kennedy's sister has taken over most of the housekeeping responsibilities. She says that she is currently able to keep up with everything but is concerned about whether she will be able to continue to care for her sister as her condition worsens.

▪ Chapter Post-test

MULTIPLE CHOICE

_____ 1. The nurse is preparing to examine the sinuses of an adult client. After examining the frontal sinuses, the nurse should proceed to examine the

A. ethmoidal sinuses.

B. laryngeal sinuses.

C. maxillary sinuses.

D. sphenoidal sinuses.

_____ 2. An adult client visits the clinic complaining of recurrent ulcers in the mouth. The nurse assesses the client's mouth and observes a painful ulcer. The nurse should document the presence of

A. a cancerous lesion.

B. *Candida albicans* infection.

C. an oral ulceration.

D. aphthous stomatitis.

_____ 3. A nurse assesses the mouth of an adult male client and observes a rough, crusty, eroded area. The nurse should

    A. refer the client for further evaluation.

    B. document the presence of herpes simplex.

    C. ask the client if his gums bleed.

    D. document the presence of a canker sore.

_____ 4. An adult client visits the clinic and tells the nurse that she has been experiencing frequent nosebleeds for the past month. The nurse should

    A. ask the client if she has had recent oral surgery.

    B. assess the client's nasal passages for blockage.

    C. ask the client if she is a smoker.

    D. refer the client for further evaluation.

_____ 5. The nurse is assessing the mouth of an older adult and observes that the client appears to have poorly fitting dentures. The nurse should instruct the client that she may be at greater risk for

    A. aspiration.

    B. malocclusion.

    C. gingivitis.

    D. throat soreness.

_____ 6. An adolescent client tells the nurse that her mother says she grinds her teeth when she sleeps. The nurse should explain to the client that grinding the teeth may be a sign of

    A. precancerous lesions.

    B. poor oral hygiene.

    C. malabsorption.

    D. stress and anxiety.

_____ 7. The nurse is planning a presentation to a group of high school students about the risk factors for oral cancer. Which of the following should be included in the nurse's plan?

    A. Diets low in fruits and vegetables are a possible risk factor for oral cancer.

    B. About 40 percent of all cancers occur in the lips, mouth, and tongue.

    C. The incidence of oral cancers is higher in women than in men.

    D. Most oral cancers are detected in people in their 70s.

_____ 8. Before examining the mouth of an adult client, the nurse should first

    A. ask the client to leave dentures in place.

    B. don sterile gloves for the procedure.

    C. offer the client mouthwash.

    D. don clean gloves for the procedure.

_____ 9. A client visits the clinic and tells the nurse that she has painful cracking in the corners of her lips. The nurse should assess the client's diet for a deficiency of

    A. vitamin C.

    B. fluoride.

    C. vitamin A.

    D. riboflavin.

_____ 10. The nurse is assessing a client who has been taking antibiotics for an infection for 10 days. The nurse observes whitish, curd-like patches in the client's mouth. The nurse should explain to the client that these spots are most likely

   A. *Candida albicans* infection.

   B. Koplik's spots.

   C. leukoplakia.

   D. Fordyce spots.

_____ 11. The nurse is assessing an adult client's oral cavity for possible oral cancer. The nurse should explain to the client that the most common site of oral cancer is the

   A. area on top of the tongue.

   B. area underneath the tongue.

   C. inside of the cheeks.

   D. area near the salivary glands.

_____ 12. The nurse is planning to inspect an adult client's mouth, using a tongue depressor. The nurse should plan to

   A. depress the tongue blade slightly off center.

   B. depress the tongue blade as close to the center as possible.

   C. ask the client to keep the mouth partially open.

   D. insert the tongue blade at the back of the client's tongue.

_____ 13. An adult client visits the clinic complaining of a sore throat. After assessing the throat, the nurse documents the client's tonsils as 4+. The nurse should explain to the client that 4+ tonsils are present when the nurse observes tonsils that are

   A. touching the uvula.

   B. visible upon inspection.

   C. touching each other.

   D. midway between the tonsillar pillars and uvula.

_____ 14. The nurse is preparing to inspect the nose of an adult client with an otoscope. The nurse plans to

   A. position the handle of the otoscope to one side.

   B. tip the client's head as far back as possible.

   C. direct the otoscope tip quickly back and down the nostril.

   D. position the handle of the otoscope straight and up.

_____ 15. The nurse has assessed the nose of an adult client and has explained to the client about her thick yellowish nasal discharge. The nurse determines that the client understands the instructions when the client says that the yellowish discharge is most likely due to

   A. too much smoking.

   B. chronic allergies.

   C. trauma to the nasal passages.

   D. an upper respiratory infection.

MATCHING

Match the terms in the left column with the correct descriptions in the right column.

Term	Description
_____ 1. Transillumination	A. Press up with thumbs on sinuses
_____ 2. Palpation and percussion	B. Touch the uvula
_____ 3. Kiesselbach's area	C. Most common site of tongue cancer
_____ 4. Stensen's ducts	D. Cracking at the corner of the lips seen in riboflavin deficiency
_____ 5. Wharton's ducts	E. Method used to test for fluid in the sinuses
_____ 6. Side of tongue	F. Sinus filled with air
_____ 7. Torus palatinus	G. Inspection using otoscope with short, wide, tip attachment
_____ 8. Bifid uvula	H. Methods used to test for sinus tenderness
_____ 9. Grade 3+ tonsils	I. Press up on brow on each side of nose
_____ 10. Method for assessing the internal nose	J. Openings found on buccal mucosa across from second upper molars
_____ 11. Method used to palpate frontal sinuses	K. Bony protuberance in the midline of the hard palate
_____ 12. Method used to palpate maxillary sinuses	L. Sinus filled with fluid or pus
_____ 13. Significance of a red glow with transillumination	M. Common site of nasal bleeding
_____ 14. Absence of a red glow with transillumination	N. A variation that looks split or partially severed and may be associated with a submucous cleft palate
_____ 15. Cheilosis	O. Normal variation that occurs in the crease between the upper and lower lip
_____ 16. Lip pits	P. Openings found on either side of the frenulum of the floor of the mouth

■ Self-Reflection and Evaluation of Learner Objectives

After you have read Chapter 13 and completed the above quizzes and activities, please identify to what degree you have met each of the following chapter learning objectives. For those objectives that you have met partially or not at all, you will want to review chapter content for that learning objective.

Objective	Very much	Somewhat	Not at all
1. Describe the structure and functions of the mouth, throat, nose, and sinuses.			
2. Discuss risk factors for cancer of the oral cavity and ways to reduce these factors.			
3. Discuss the prevalence of oral cavity cancer across cultures.			
4. Obtain an accurate nursing history of the client's mouth, throat, nose, and sinuses.			
5. Explain how to prepare the client for an examination of the mouth, throat, nose, and sinuses.			
6. Describe the equipment necessary to perform this assessment.			
7. Describe the two physical exam techniques (inspection and palpation) used for this assessment.			
8. Inspect the lips, buccal mucosa, gums, and tongue for color and consistency, lesions, ulcers, or induration, noting Stensen's ducts, Wharton's ducts, and breath odor.			
9. Inspect the teeth for number, color, condition, and alignment.			
10. Inspect the throat for characteristics and position of the uvula, presence of gag reflex, grading of the tonsils, and tonsil and palate for color, size, condition, exudates, or lesions.			
11. Assess the nose for internal and external color, shape, consistence, tenderness, smell, and patency of airflow.			
12. Inspect the turbinates for color, moisture, and lesions.			
13. Describe the three physical exam techniques (palpation, percussion, and transillumination) used to assess the sinuses.			
14. Inspect the sinuses for tenderness, air versus fluid, or pus filling.			
15. Describe cultural variations of the mouth and throat.			
16. Describe expected changes with aging of the mouth, throat, nose, and sinuses.			

For additional information on this book, be sure to visit *http://connection.lww.com*.

Thoracic and Lung Assessment

CHAPTER OVERVIEW

Respiration is a life-sustaining function, which makes precise assessment of the chest and breathing structures an essential nursing skill. Use the following exercises and quizzes as a guide to effective physical assessment of the thorax and lungs.

■ Chapter Pretest

MULTIPLE CHOICE

_____ 1. The clavicles extend from the acromion of the scapula to the part of the sternum termed the

    A. body.

    B. xiphoid process.

    C. angle.

    D. manubrium.

_____ 2. A bony ridge located at the point where the manubrium articulates with the body of the sternum is termed the sternal

    A. angle.

    B. notch.

    C. space.

    D. prominens.

_____ 3. The spinous process termed the vertebra prominens is which cervical vertebra?

    A. Fifth.

    B. Sixth.

    C. Seventh.

    D. Eighth.

_____ 4. The apex of each lung is located at the

    A. level of the diaphragm.

    B. area slightly above the clavicle.

    C. level of the sixth rib.

    D. left oblique fissure.

_____ 5. The thin, double-layered serous membrane that lines the chest cavity is termed
   A. parietal pleura.
   B. pulmonary pleura.
   C. visceral pleura.
   D. thoracic pleura.

_____ 6. The lining of the trachea and bronchi, which serves to remove dust, foreign bodies, and bacteria, is termed the
   A. bronchioles.
   B. alveolar sacs.
   C. alveolar ducts.
   D. cilia.

_____ 7. Under normal circumstances, the strongest stimulus in a human being to breathe is
   A. hypoxemia.
   B. hypocapnia.
   C. pH changes.
   D. hypercapnia.

LABELING ACTIVITY

Label the following structures of the anterior thoracic cage.

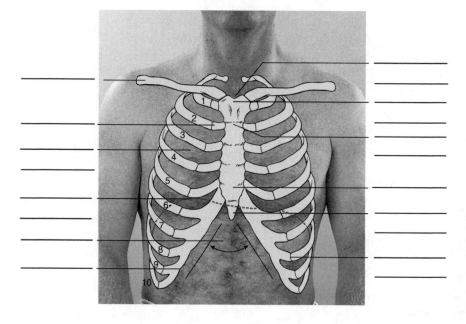

Anterior thoracic cage.

Label the structure indicated by the line; then match your answer with the label on the matching figure in chapter 14 of your textbook.

Label the following structures of the posterior thoracic cage.

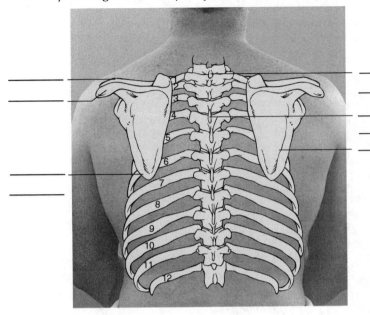

Posterior thoracic cage.

Label the structure indicated by the line; then match your answer with the label on the matching figure in chapter 14 of your textbook.

Label the following structures of the anterior vertical lines.

Anterior vertical lines.

Label the structure indicated by the line; then match your answer with the label on the matching figure in chapter 14 of your textbook.

Label the following structures of the posterior vertical lines.

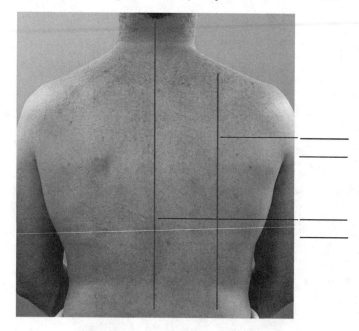

Posterior vertical lines.

Label the structure indicated by the line; then match your answer with the label on the matching figure in chapter 14 of your textbook.

Label the following structures of the lateral vertical lines.

Lateral vertical lines.

Label the structure indicated by the line; then match your answer with the label on the matching figure in chapter 14 of your textbook.

■ Learner Activities

1. Review the information in the Risk Factors display in Chapter 14 of *Health Assessment in Nursing*, 2nd edition. Determine your own risk for lung cancer. Next, identify ethnic groups that are at highest risk for lung cancer.

2. Find an elderly client, friend or relative who will let you examine his or her thorax and lungs. Discuss with peers your findings as they compare with the findings in a younger person's thorax and lungs.

INTERVIEWING AND RECORDING ASSESSMENT FINDINGS

Use the following Nursing History Checklist as your guide to interviewing and recording your findings in thoracic and lung assessment.

NURSING HISTORY CHECKLIST

Questions	Satisfactory data	Needs additional data	Data missing
Current Symptoms			
1. Difficulty breathing (at rest, with specific activities, while sleeping, other symptoms when having trouble breathing)?			
2. Chest pain associated with a cold, a fever, or deep breathing?			
3. Cough, with or without sputum?			
Past History			
1. Prior respiratory problems?			
2. Previous thoracic surgery, biopsy, or trauma?			
3. Allergies, symptoms/treatments?			
4. Pulmonary studies/tests: chest x-ray, TB skin test, or influenza immunization?			
Family History			
1. Family history of lung disease?			
Lifestyle and Health Practices			
1. Use of tobacco products, cigarettes or cigars (number of years, number per day)?			
2. Exposure to environmental conditions that affect breathing at work or at home, including secondhand smoke?			
3. Difficulty performing usual daily activities?			
4. Degree of stress, effect on breathing?			
5. Medications for breathing (prescribed or OTC), other breathing treatments?			

PERFORMING PHYSICAL ASSESSMENT

Use the following Physical Assessment Checklist as your guide to performing a thoracic and lung assessment.

PHYSICAL ASSESSMENT CHECKLIST

Assessment Skill	Findings (Normal or Abnormal) and Notes		Performance (Satisfactory, Needs Improvement, Unsatisfactory)		
	N	A	S	N	U
1. Gather equipment (gown and drape, gloves, stethoscope, exam light, mask, skin marker, metric ruler).	☐	☐	☐	☐	☐
2. Explain procedure to client.	☐	☐	☐	☐	☐
3. Ask client to put on a gown.	☐	☐	☐	☐	☐
Posterior Thorax					
1. Inspect for shape and configuration of the chest wall and position of scapulae.	☐	☐	☐	☐	☐
2. Inspect for use of accessory muscles.	☐	☐	☐	☐	☐
3. Inspect client's positioning, noting posture and ability to support weight while breathing.	☐	☐	☐	☐	☐
4. Palpate for tenderness and sensation with gloved fingers.	☐	☐	☐	☐	☐
5. Palpate for surface characteristics such as lesions or masses with gloved fingers.	☐	☐	☐	☐	☐
6. Palpate for fremitus, using the ball or ulnar edge of one hand while client says "ninety-nine." Assess for symmetry and intensity of vibration.	☐	☐	☐	☐	☐
7. Palpate for chest expansion. Place hands on the posterior chest wall with your thumbs at the level of T9 or T10, and observe the movement of your thumbs as the client takes a deep breath.	☐	☐	☐	☐	☐
8. Percuss for tone, starting at the apices above the scapulae and across the tops of both shoulders.	☐	☐	☐	☐	☐
9. Percuss intercostal spaces across and down, comparing sides.	☐	☐	☐	☐	☐
10. Percuss to the lateral aspects at the bases of the lungs, and compare sides.	☐	☐	☐	☐	☐
11. Percuss for diaphragmatic excursion, using the procedure on text page 265.	☐	☐	☐	☐	☐
12. Auscultate for breath sounds (normal: bronchial, bronchiovesicular, and vesicular), noting location.	☐	☐	☐	☐	☐
13. Auscultate for adventitious sounds (crackles, fine or course, pleural friction rub, wheeze, sibilant or sonorous).	☐	☐	☐	☐	☐
14. Auscultate for voice sounds over the chest wall: Bronchophony-ask client to repeat the phrase "ninety-nine."					
Egophony-ask the client to repeat the letter "E."	☐	☐	☐	☐	☐
Whispered pectoriloquy-ask the client to whisper the phrase "one-two-three."					

PHYSICAL ASSESSMENT CHECKLIST

Assessment Skill	Findings (Normal or Abnormal) and Notes		Performance (Satisfactory, Needs Improvement, Unsatisfactory)		
	N	A	S	N	U
Anterior Thorax					
1. Inspect for shape and configuration to determine the ratio of anteroposterior diameter to transverse diameter (normally 1:2).	☐	☐	☐	☐	☐
2. Inspect for position of sternum from anterior and lateral viewpoints.	☐	☐	☐	☐	☐
3. Inspect for slope of the ribs from anterior and lateral viewpoints.	☐	☐	☐	☐	☐
4. Inspect for quality and pattern of respiration, noting breathing characteristics, rate, rhythm, and depth.	☐	☐	☐	☐	☐
5. Inspect intercostal spaces while client breathes normally.	☐	☐	☐	☐	☐
6. Inspect for use of accessory muscles.	☐	☐	☐	☐	☐
7. Palpate for tenderness and sensation, using fingers.	☐	☐	☐	☐	☐
8. Palpate surface characteristics such as lesions or masses, using fingers of gloved hand.	☐	☐	☐	☐	☐
9. Palpate for fremitus while the client says "ninety-nine."	☐	☐	☐	☐	☐
10. Palpate for chest expansion by placing hands on the anterolateral wall with the thumbs along the costal margins and pointing toward the xiphoid process. Observe movement of the thumbs as the client takes a deep breath.	☐	☐	☐	☐	☐
11. Percuss for tone above the clavicles and then the intercostal spaces across and down, comparing sides.	☐	☐	☐	☐	☐
12. Auscultate for breath sounds, adventitious sounds, and voice sounds.	☐	☐	☐	☐	☐
Analysis of Data					
1. Formulate nursing diagnoses (wellness, risk, actual).	☐	☐	☐	☐	☐
2. Formulate collaborative problems.	☐	☐	☐	☐	☐
3. Make necessary referrals.	☐	☐	☐	☐	☐

■ Chapter Post-test

MULTIPLE CHOICE

_____ 1. While assessing an adult client, the client tells the nurse that she "has had difficulty catching her breath since yesterday." The nurse should assess the client further for signs and symptoms of

A. emphysema.

B. cardiac disease.

C. trauma to the chest.

D. infection.

_____ 2. An adult client visits the clinic and tells the nurse that he has been "spitting up rust-colored sputum." The nurse should refer the client to the physician for possible

   A. pulmonary edema.

   B. bronchitis.

   C. asthma.

   D. tuberculosis.

_____ 3. The nurse is planning a presentation to a group of high school students on the topic of lung cancer. Which of the following should the nurse plan to include in the presentation?

   A. Compared with whites in the United States, African Americans have a lower incidence of lung cancer.

   B. Lung cancer is the third leading cause of death in the United States.

   C. There is a higher incidence of lung cancer in women than men in the United States.

   D. Studies have indicated that there is a genetic component in the development of lung cancer.

_____ 4. While assessing an adult client, the nurse observes decreased chest expansion at the bases of the client's lungs. The nurse should refer the client to a physician for possible

   A. atelectasis.

   B. pneumonia.

   C. chest trauma.

   D. chronic obstructive pulmonary disease.

_____ 5. The nurse is planning to percuss the chest of an adult male client for diaphragmatic excursion. The nurse should begin the assessment by

   A. asking the client to take a deep breath and hold it.

   B. percussing upward from the base of the lungs.

   C. percussing downward until the tone changes to resonance.

   D. asking the client to exhale forcefully and hold his breath.

_____ 6. The nurse is preparing to auscultate the posterior thorax of an adult female client. The nurse should

   A. place the bell of the stethoscope firmly on the posterior chest wall.

   B. auscultate from the base of the lungs to the apices.

   C. ask the client to breathe deeply through her mouth.

   D. ask the client to breathe normally through her nose.

_____ 7. While assessing the thoracic area of an adult client, the nurse plans to auscultate for voice sounds. To assess bronchophony, the nurse should ask the client to

   A. repeat the phrase "ninety-nine."

   B. repeat the letter "E."

   C. whisper the phrase "one-two-three."

   D. repeat the letter "A."

_____ 8. The nurse assesses an adult client's thoracic area and observes a markedly sunken sternum and adjacent cartilages. The nurse should document the client's

A. pectus thorax.

B. pectus excavatum.

C. pectus carinatum.

D. pectus diaphragm.

_____ 9. The nurse assesses an adult client and observes that the client's breathing pattern is very labored and noisy, with occasional coughing. The nurse should refer the client to a physician for possible

A. chronic bronchitis.

B. atelectasis.

C. renal failure.

D. congestive heart failure.

_____ 10. While assessing an adult client's lungs during the postoperative period, the nurse detects coarse crackles. The nurse should refer the client to a physician for possible

A. pneumonia.

B. pleuritis.

C. bronchitis.

D. asthma.

_____ 11. The nurse assesses an adult client's breath sounds and hears sonorous wheezes, primarily during the client's expiration. The nurse should refer the client to a physician for possible

A. asthma.

B. chronic emphysema.

C. pleuritis.

D. bronchitis.

_____ 12. The nurse has assessed the respiratory pattern of an adult client. The nurse determines that the client is exhibiting Kussmaul's respirations with hyperventilation. The nurse should contact the client's physician because this type of respiratory pattern usually indicates

A. diabetic ketoacidosis.

B. central nervous system injury.

C. drug overdose.

D. congestive heart failure.

MATCHING

Match the terms in the left column with the correct description in the right column.

Term	Description
____ 1. Promotes the strongest stimulus to breathe	A. High-pitched, short, popping sounds
____ 2. Orthopnea	B. Forward protrusion of the sternum
____ 3. Crepitus	C. High-pitched, musical sounds
____ 4. Pectus excavatum	D. An increase in carbon dioxide in the blood
____ 5. Pectus carinatum	E. Low-pitched, bubbling, moist sounds
____ 6. Pleural friction rub	F. Low-pitched snoring or moaning sounds
____ 7. Wheeze (sibilant)	G. Difficulty breathing when lying supine
____ 8. Wheeze (sonorous)	H. Markedly sunken sternum and adjacent cartilage
____ 9. Crackles (fine)	I. Low-pitched, dry grating sounds
____ 10. Crackles (coarse)	J. A "crackling" sensation

CRITICAL THINKING AND CASE STUDIES

1. Read the following case study. Develop appropriate nursing diagnoses for the client.

Bo Thomson, 61, arrives at the outpatient clinic complaining of shortness of breath. He tells you that he has been employed by an asbestos removal company for the past 15 years. He says he has followed safety precautions "most of the time." He also tells you that on weekends he always relaxes by drinking beer and smoking a little at his favorite bar. He is divorced and has two grown sons, who live about 20 miles away. There is no history of lung cancer in his family that he can remember. He says, "I know I don't live a very healthy life, but I'm too old to change my ways now."

2. On the basis of the following assessment information, work through the steps of analyzing the data. Identify abnormal data and strengths in **subjective and objective findings**, assemble **cue clusters**, draw **inferences**, make possible **nursing diagnoses**, identify **defining characteristics**, **confirm or rule out** the nursing diagnosis, and **document** your conclusions.

   Use the blank diagnostic analysis charts provided at the end of this book to guide your thinking. You may want to write on the chart or use separate paper. Propose nursing diagnoses that are specific to the client in the case study. Identify collaborative problems, if any, for this client. Finally, identify data, if any, that point toward a medical problem requiring a referral.

Theresa Johnson is a 55-year-old white woman. She is a part-time secretary for a local businessman and is very active in her community. She is married and has two children. T.J. presents at the nursing clinic this morning with a complaint of extreme shortness of breath. When entering the examination room, she appears very anxious and states that she has experienced this problem since yesterday afternoon.

Theresa has no previous diagnosis of asthma, allergies, or respiratory problems, but her brother and father have cases of mild asthma. The client has smoked for 35 years but reports limiting her smoking to a pack every 2 to 3 days for the past 10 years. Before that, she reports having smoked a pack every day. She worked in her office yesterday and reports having felt fine. She met friends at a local park for lunch but denies anything unusual about her daily activity. She states she has experienced "tightness in my chest," increasing in severity since about 5:00 p.m. yesterday. She denies any other associated symptoms such as pain or cough. Her discomfort made sleeping difficult last night, and she states that she hasn't eaten today because of her shortness of breath.

She currently takes no medications. She reports having no regular exercise program but denies any intolerance to activity until the onset of dyspnea. She reports having tried only rest to alleviate the problem and knows "nothing else to do but go to the doctor.'

Her respiratory rate is 26 breaths/minute and appears somewhat labored. The client seems somewhat apprehensive and experiences obvious dyspnea on even mild exertion. Her anteroposterior diameter is within normal limits. The use of accessory muscles is noted, with respiration immediately after exertion. Expiration is somewhat labored and prolonged. Tactile fremitus is decreased, especially in lower lobes. Percussion tones are resonant over all lung fields. Breath sounds are decreased, with prolonged expiration. Voice sounds are also decreased. Expiratory wheeze is noted throughout the lung fields, especially bilaterally in the lower lobes.

■ Self-Reflection and Evaluation of Learning Objectives

After you have read Chapter 14 and completed the above quizzes and activities, please identify to what degree you have met each of the following chapter learning objectives. For those objectives that you have met partially or not at all, you will want to review chapter content for that learning objective.

Objective	Very much	Somewhat	Not at all
1. Describe the structures and functions of the thorax and lungs.			
2. Discuss risk factors for lung cancer and ways to reduce these risk factors.			
3. Discuss the prevalence of lung cancer across the cultures.			
4. Obtain an accurate nursing history of the client's thorax and lungs.			
5. Explain how to prepare the client for an examination of the thorax and lungs.			
6. Inspect the client's chest for shape and configuration of the chest wall and position of the scapulae.			

(continues)

(Continued)

Objective	Very much	Somewhat	Not at all
7. Inspect the client's use of accessory muscles during respirations.			
8. Inspect the client's positioning.			
9. Palpate the client's thorax for tenderness and sensation, surface characteristics, fremitus, and chest expansion.			
10. Percuss the client's thorax for tone and diaphragmatic excursion.			
11. Describe expected age-related changes of the thorax and lungs.			
12. Assess the client's breath sounds by auscultating the lungs.			
13. Distinguish between normal and abnormal breath sounds.			
14. Auscultate the client's posterior chest for adventitious sounds.			
15. Auscultate the client's posterior chest for voice sounds.			
16. Inspect the client's anterior chest for shape and configuration, position of the sternum, and slope of the ribs.			
17. Inspect the client's respirations for quality and pattern.			
18. Inspect the client's intercostal spaces and use of accessory muscles.			
19. Palpate the anterior chest for tenderness and sensation and surface characteristics.			
20. Palpate the anterior chest for fremitus and chest expansion.			
21. Percuss the anterior chest.			
22. Auscultate the anterior chest for breath sounds, adventitious sounds, and voice sounds.			
23. Auscultate the client's posterior chest for adventitious sounds.			

For additional information on this book, be sure to visit *http://connection.lww.com.*

CHAPTER 15

Breast and Lymphatic Assessment

CHAPTER OVERVIEW

Breast and lymphatic health is an important issue, not only for women during their childbearing years and throughout their lives, but also for men, whose breast development and health may be affected by various factors such as medications and hormonal problems. Use the following exercises and quizzes to guide your physical assessment of the breast and lymphatic structures.

■ Chapter Pretest

MULTIPLE CHOICE

_____ 1. At puberty, the female breasts enlarge in response to estrogen and

   A. progesterone.

   B. aldosterone.

   C. lactogen.

   D. prolactin.

_____ 2. Elevated sebaceous glands, known as Montgomery's glands, are located in the breast's

   A. nipples.

   B. hair follicles.

   C. lactiferous ducts.

   D. areolas.

_____ 3. The functional part of the breast that allows for milk production consists of tissue termed

   A. fibrous.

   B. glandular.

   C. adipose.

   D. lactiferous.

_____ 4. Fibrous tissue that provides support for the glandular tissue of the breasts is termed

   A. lateral ligaments.

   B. Wharton's ligaments.

   C. pectoral ligaments.

   D. Cooper's ligaments.

_____ 5. The size and shape of the breasts in females is related to the amount of
   A. glandular tissue.
   B. fibrous tissue.
   C. lactiferous ducts.
   D. fatty tissue.

_____ 6. The lymph nodes that are responsible for drainage from the arms are the
   A. lateral lymph nodes.
   B. central lymph nodes.
   C. anterior lymph nodes.
   D. posterior lymph nodes.

LABELING ACTIVITIES

Label the following structures of the anterior chest.

Landmarks and their position in the thorax.

Label the structure indicated by the line; then match your answer with the label on the matching figure in chapter 15 of your textbook.

Label the following breast quadrants.

Breast quadrants.

Label the structure indicated by the line; then match your answer with the label on the matching figure in chapter 15 of your textbook.

Label the internal anatomic structures of the breast.

Internal anatomy of the breast.

Label the structure indicated by the line; then match your answer with the label on the matching figure in chapter 15 of your textbook.

Label the following major axillary lymph nodes.

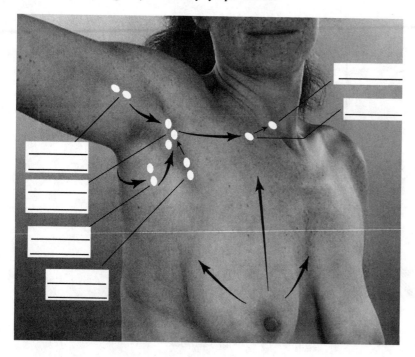

The major axillary lymph nodes.

Label the structure indicated by the line; then match your answer with the label on the matching figure in chapter 15 of your textbook.

■ Learner Activities

After reading Chapter 15, participate in the following learning activities.

1. Review the information in the Risk Factors display in Chapter 15 in your textbook. Determine your own risk of breast cancer. Next, identify ethnic groups that are at higher risk for breast cancer.

2. Use a breast model to review the anatomy and function of each anatomic structure. Discuss the changes of the breast and surrounding tissue that occur with aging.

3. Obtain an information packet from a local agency that performs mammograms. Review the material with a lab partner, and discuss how you would teach a client to do a breast self-examination.

INTERVIEWING AND RECORDING ASSESSMENT FINDINGS

Use the following Nursing History Checklist as your guide to interviewing and recording your findings in a breast assessment.

NURSING HISTORY CHECKLIST

Questions	Normal findings	Abnormal findings	Data missing
Current Symptoms			
1. Changes in breasts (lumps, swelling, redness, warmth, dimpling, size, firmness, pain, discharge)?			

NURSING HISTORY CHECKLIST

Questions	Normal findings	Abnormal findings	Data missing
Past History			
1. Previous problems with breasts (treatment and surgery)?			
2. Age at menses?			
3. Age at menopause?			
4. Given birth?			
5. Age at first birth?			
6. First and last day of menstrual cycle?			
Family History			
1. Family history of breast cancer?			
Lifestyle and Health Practices			
1. Use of hormones, contraceptives, or antidepressants?			
2. Exposure to radiation, benzene, or asbestos?			
3. Usual diet, including intake of alcohol, coffee, tea, soft drinks, and chocolate?			
4. Usual exercise patterns?			
5. Type of bra worn during exercise?			
6. Examine own breasts/frequency?			
7. Last breast exam by physician?			
8. Last mammogram?			

PERFORMING PHYSICAL ASSESSMENT

Use the following Physical Assessment Checklist as your guide to performing a breast assessment.

PHYSICAL ASSESSMENT CHECKLIST

Assessment Skill	Findings (Normal or Abnormal) and Notes		Performance (Satisfactory, Needs Improvement, Unsatisfactory)		
	N	A	S	N	U
1. Gather equipment (centimeter ruler, small pillow, gloves, client handout on breast self-examination, slide for specimen).	☐	☐	☐	☐	☐
2. Explain procedure to client.	☐	☐	☐	☐	☐
3. Ask client to put on a gown.	☐	☐	☐	☐	☐
Female Breasts					
1. *Inspect breasts*					
a. Size and symmetry	☐	☐	☐	☐	☐

(continues)

PHYSICAL ASSESSMENT CHECKLIST *(Continued)*

Assessment Skill	Findings (Normal or Abnormal) and Notes		Performance (Satisfactory, Needs Improvement, Unsatisfactory)		
	N	A	S	N	U
b. Color and texture	☐	☐	☐	☐	☐
c. Superficial venous patterns	☐	☐	☐	☐	☐
d. Retraction and dimpling	☐	☐	☐	☐	☐
e. Bilaterally, note color, size, shape, and texture of areolas	☐	☐	☐	☐	☐
f. Bilaterally, note size and direction of nipples	☐	☐	☐	☐	☐
2. *Palpate breasts*					
a. Texture and elasticity	☐	☐	☐	☐	☐
b. Tenderness and temperature	☐	☐	☐	☐	☐
c. Masses: noting location, size in centimeters, shape, mobility, consistency, and tenderness	☐	☐	☐	☐	☐
d. Palpate nipples by compressing nipple gently between thumb and index finger; observe for discharge	☐	☐	☐	☐	☐
e. Palpate mastectomy site, if applicable, observing the scar and any remaining breast or axillary tissue for redness, lesions, lumps, swelling, or tenderness	☐	☐	☐	☐	☐
Male Breasts					
1. Inspect and palpate the breasts, areolas, and nipples for swelling, nodules, or ulcerations.	☐	☐	☐	☐	☐
Axillae					
1. Inspect for rashes or infection.	☐	☐	☐	☐	☐
2. Hold the elbow with one hand and use the three fingerpads of your other hand to palpate firmly the axillary lymph nodes.	☐	☐	☐	☐	☐
3. Palpate high into the axillae, moving downward against the ribs to feel for the central nodes. Continue down the posterior axillae to feel for the posterior nodes.	☐	☐	☐	☐	☐
4. Use bimanual palpation to feel for the anterior axillary nodes.	☐	☐	☐	☐	☐
5. Palpate down the inner aspect of the upper arm.	☐	☐	☐	☐	☐
Analysis of Data					
1. Formulate nursing diagnoses (wellness, risk, actual).	☐	☐	☐	☐	☐
2. Formulate collaborative problems.	☐	☐	☐	☐	☐
3. Make necessary referrals.	☐	☐	☐	☐	☐

CRITICAL THINKING AND CASE STUDIES

1. Read the following case study and analyze the client's risk factors for the development of breast cancer.

   Julia Hershey is a 67-year-old retired secretary. Her mother and a sister have been treated for breast cancer, but Ms. Hershey has no personal history of cancer. She gave birth to her only child when she was 37 years of age. She states that her daughter was a "bottle baby" and that breast-feeding was not "proper" back when her daughter was a baby. Ms. Hershey states that she went through the "change" (menopause) in her late 40s. Although she understands how to perform breast self-examinations, Ms. Hershey states that she does not do them on a regular basis. Her chart indicates that her last mammogram was 6 years ago.

2. Explain how you would assess the male breast and surrounding tissue. What would you explain to the male client about this part of the examination?

3. On the basis of the following assessment information, work through the steps of analyzing the data. Identify abnormal data and strengths in **subjective** and **objective findings.** Assemble **cue clusters,** draw **inferences,** make possible **nursing diagnoses,** identify **defining characteristics, confirm** or **rule out** the nursing diagnosis, and **document** your conclusions. Use the blank diagnostic analysis charts provided at the end of this book to guide your thinking. You may want to write on the chart or use separate paper. Propose nursing diagnoses that are specific to the client in the case study. Identify collaborative problems, if any, for this client. Finally, identify data, if any, that point toward a medical problem requiring a referral.

Carol Lawrence, a teacher, is a 42-year-old white woman. She is married and has three children. She has a history of fibrocystic breast disease. She felt a distinct tender lump in her left breast while taking a shower 2 days ago. At age 56, the client's mother died of breast cancer. Carol had one breast biopsy years ago, and the results were negative for cancer. At that time her mammography revealed fibrocystic breast disease. Carol has one natural child, aged 4 years, and two adopted children, aged 10 and 12 years. She states, "I'm so afraid that this might be cancer."

Physical examination reveals symmetric, round, smooth, pink breasts. The areolae are dark brown, and the nipples are everted. No rashes, lesions, dimpling, or retraction of breast tissue are noted while the client is in various positions. The client has tears in her eyes and a quavering voice. Palpation reveals generalized bilateral breast tenderness. Clear discharge is excreted from the left nipple. Bilateral, multiple, scattered, small, rubbery nodules are palpated bilaterally. No enlarged lumps or masses are palpated in the right breast. A 3 centimeter × 2 centimeter × 1 centimeter firm, oval, nonmobile, tender lump is palpated in left breast. No lymph nodes are palpable. Demonstrates appropriate technique for breast self-examination.

DISPLAY 15-1. Breast Self-Examination (BSE)

STEP 1

1. Stand before a mirror.
2. Check both breasts for anything unusual.
3. Look for discharge from the nipple, puckering, dimpling, or scaling of the skin.

The next two steps are done to check for any changes in the contour of your breasts. As you do them, you should be able to feel your muscles tighten.

STEP 3

1. Next, press your hands firmly on your hips and bow slightly toward the mirror as you pull your shoulders and elbows forward.
2. Note any change in the contour of your breasts.

Some women do the next part of the examination in the shower. Your fingers will glide easily over soapy skin, so you can concentrate on feeling for changes inside the breast.

STEP 2

1. Watch closely in the mirror as you clasp your hands behind your head and press your hands forward.
2. Note any change in the contour of your breasts.

STEP 4

1. Raise your left arm.
2. Use three or four fingers of your right hand to feel your left breast firmly, carefully, and thoroughly.
3. Beginning at the outer edge, press the flat part of your fingers in small circles, moving the circles slowly around the breast.
4. Gradually work toward the nipple.
5. Be sure to examine the whole breast.
6. Pay special attention to the area between the breast and the underarm, including the underarm itself.
7. Feel for any unusual lumps or masses under the skin.

STEP 5
1. Gently squeeze the nipple and look for a discharge.
2. If you have any discharge during the month-whether or not it is during your BSE-see your doctor.
3. Repeat the examination on your right breast.

STEP 6
1. Steps 4 and 5 should be repeated lying down.
2. Lie flat on your back with your left arm over your head and a pillow or folded towel under your left shoulder. (This position flattens your breast and makes it easier to check.)
3. Use the same circular motion described above.
4. Repeat on your right breast.

■ Chapter Post-test

MULTIPLE CHOICE

_____ 1. After assessing the breasts of a female client, the nurse should explain to the client that most breast tumors occur in the

    A. upper inner quadrant.

    B. lower inner quadrant.

    C. upper outer quadrant.

    D. lower outer quadrant.

_____ 2. A female client tells the nurse that her breasts become lumpy and sore before menstruation but get better at the end of the menstrual cycle. The nurse should explain to the client that these symptoms are often associated with

    A. malignant tumors.

    B. fibroadenoma.

    C. fibrocystic breast disease.

    D. increased estrogen production.

_____ 3. The nurse has discussed the risks for breast cancer with a group of high school seniors. The nurse determines that one of the students needs further instructions when the student says that one risk factor is

    A. having a baby before the age of 20 years.

    B. a family history of breast cancer.

    C. consumption of a high-fat diet.

    D. late menopause.

_____ 4. Cultural beliefs about the causes of breast cancer do not always agree with medical findings. Hispanic Americans often associate breast cancer with

   A. improper diet.

   B. punishment from God.

   C. physical stress.

   D. evil thoughts.

_____ 5. The nurse is working with a community group to set up teaching programs to increase awareness among African-American women about preventive screening techniques for breast cancer. In the teaching program, the nurse should plan to include

   A. local female physicians who work with cancer clients.

   B. hospital clinic workers from various racial backgrounds.

   C. nurses who work in outpatient centers.

   D. breast cancer patients of the same race.

_____ 6. The nurse is caring for an adult female client when the client tells the nurse that she has had a clear discharge from her nipples for the past month. The nurse should ask the client if she has been taking

   A. antidepressants.

   B. antibiotics.

   C. insulin.

   D. contraceptives.

_____ 7. The nurse is assessing an adult male client when the nurse observes gynecomastia in the client. The nurse should ask the client if he is taking any medications for

   A. inflammation.

   B. depression.

   C. infection.

   D. ulcers.

_____ 8. The nurse is caring for a female client who has received a diagnosis of fibrocystic breast disease. The nurse has instructed the client about the disease. The nurse determines that the client needs further instructions when the client says she should avoid drinking

   A. regular coffee.

   B. regular tea.

   C. diet colas.

   D. grapefruit juice.

_____ 9. The nurse plans to instruct an adult female client with regular menstrual cycles, who is not taking oral contraceptives, about breast self-examination. The nurse should plan to instruct the client to perform breast self-examination

   A. during menstruation.

   B. on the same day every month.

   C. midway between the cycles.

   D. right after menstruation.

_____ 10. The nurse observes an orange-peel appearance, or peau d'orange, of the areolae of a client's breasts. The nurse should explain to the client that this is most likely due to

A. blocked lymphatic drainage.

B. fibrocystic breast disease.

C. fibroadenomas.

D. radiation therapy.

_____ 11. The nurse is assessing a 50-year-old client's breasts and observes a spontaneous discharge of fluid from the left nipple. The nurse should

A. document this as a normal finding.

B. ask the client if she has had retracted nipples.

C. refer the client for a cytology examination.

D. determine whether the client wears a supportive bra.

_____ 12. The nurse observes dimpling in an adult female client's breasts. The nurse should explain to the client that dimpling of the breast may indicate a

A. fibroadenoma.

B. tumor.

C. genetic deviation.

D. fibrocystic breast.

_____ 13. The nurse is preparing to examine the breasts of a female client who had a left radical mastectomy 3 years ago. When examining the client, the nurse observes redness at the scar area. The nurse should explain to the client that this may be indicative of

A. additional tumors.

B. poor lymphatic drainage.

C. an infectious process.

D. metastasis to the right breast.

_____ 14. A client has had a recent mastectomy and visits the clinic for postoperative evaluation. The client tells the nurse that she has been depressed and feels as if she is no longer a woman. The most appropriate nursing diagnosis for this client is

A. Ineffective individual coping related to mastectomy.

B. Fear of additional breast cancer related to presence of risk factors.

C. PC: Hematoma after mastectomy.

D. disturbed body image related to mastectomy.

MATCHING

Match the terms in the left column with the correct descriptions in the right column.

Term	Description
_____ 1. Axillary lymph nodes	A. Lymphatic obstruction, causing edema, which thickens the skin, exaggerates the hair follicles, and gives the breast an orange-peel or pigskin look
_____ 2. Mammary gland	
_____ 3. Mastectomy	B. Darkly pigmented area surrounding the nipple of the mammary gland
_____ 4. Lactiferous duct	C. Enlargement of one or both male breasts, seen more frequently in adolescent boys and elderly men
_____ 5. Lactiferous sinus	D. Reservoirs for storing milk, located behind the nipple
_____ 6. Cooper's ligaments	E. Pigmented projection at the tip of each breast, which allows passage of milk from the breast
_____ 7. Tail of Spence	F. Specialized gland of the skin of females, which secretes milk for nourishment of the young
_____ 8. Areola	
_____ 9. Nipple	G. Roentgenography of the breast to detect any underlying mass
_____ 10. Paget's disease	H. Ducts conveying the milk secreted by the lobes of the breast to and through the nipples
_____ 11. Peau d'orange	I. Groups of lymph nodes located under the arm (the axilla)
_____ 12. Mastitis	J. Inflammation of the breast
_____ 13. Mammography	K. Cone-shaped breast tissue that projects up into the axillae
_____ 14. Gynecomastia	L. Surgical removal of breast tissue
	M. Fibrous glands extending vertically from the breast surface to attach on the chest wall muscles
	N. Erythematous scaling lesion of the breast, involving the nipple and areola unilaterally, and associated with an underlying malignancy

■ Self-Reflection and Evaluation of Learning Objectives

After you have read Chapter 15 and completed the above quizzes and activities, please identify to what degree you have met each of the following chapter learning objectives. For those objectives that you have met partially or not at all, you will want to review chapter content for that learning objective.

Objective	Very much	Somewhat	Not at all
1. Describe the structure and functions of the breast and major axillary lymph nodes.			
2. Discuss risk factors for breast cancer and ways to reduce these risk factors.			
3. Discuss the prevalence of breast cancer across cultures.			
4. Obtain an accurate nursing history of the client's breast and axillary region.			

Objective	Very much	Somewhat	Not at all
5. Explain how to prepare the client for an examination of the breasts and axillary region.			
6. Describe the equipment necessary to perform a breast and axillary assessment.			
7. Describe the two physical examination techniques (inspection and palpation) used to assess the breasts and axillae.			
8. Assess the female breasts for size, symmetry, color, texture, and venous patterns.			
9. Describe expected changes with aging of the female breasts.			
10. Assess the areolas for color, size, shape, and texture. Assess the size and direction of the nipples.			
11. Assess breasts for retraction and dimpling.			
12. Palpate the breasts for texture, elasticity, temperature, and masses.			
13. Describe the procedure for palpating the nipples and collecting a specimen.			
14. Inspect and palpate the male breasts, areolas, and nipples.			
15. Assess the axillae for rashes or infections.			
16. Teach clients how to perform breast self-examinations.			
17. Inspect the client's respirations for quality and pattern.			
18. Inspect the client's intercostal spaces and use of accessory muscles.			
19. Palpate the anterior chest for tenderness, sensation, and surface characteristics.			
20. Palpate the anterior chest for fremitus and chest expansion.			
21. Percuss the anterior chest.			
22. Auscultate the anterior chest for breath sounds, adventitious sounds, and voice sounds.			
23. Auscultate the client's posterior chest for adventitious sounds.			

For additional information on this book, be sure to visit *http://connection.lww.com.*

CHAPTER 16

Heart and Neck Vessel Assessment

CHAPTER OVERVIEW

One of the most complex and important aspects of the physical examination is the assessment of heart function and neck vessel patency. The heart needs to pump blood efficiently, and the neck vessels need to deliver the blood to and from the brain to ensure health, life, and mental and physical function. Use the following quizzes and exercises as a guide to your physical assessment activities.

■ Chapter Pretest

MULTIPLE CHOICE

Choose the one best answer for each of the following multiple-choice questions.

_____ 1. The anterior chest area that overlies the heart and great vessels is called the
  A. precordium.
  B. epicardium.
  C. myocardium.
  D. endocardium.

_____ 2. The bicuspid, or mitral, valve is located
  A. between the left atrium and the left ventricle.
  B. between the right atrium and the right ventricle.
  C. at the beginning of the ascending aorta.
  D. at the exit of each ventricle near the great vessels.

_____ 3. The semilunar valves are located
  A. at the exit of each ventricle at the beginning of the great vessels.
  B. between the right atrium and the right ventricle.
  C. between the left atrium and the left ventricle.
  D. at the beginning of the ascending aorta.

_____ 4. The sinoatrial node of the heart is located on the
  A. posterior wall of the right atrium.
  B. anterior wall of the right atrium.
  C. upper intraventricular system.
  D. anterior wall of the left atrium.

_____ 5. The P wave phase of an electrocardiogram (ECG) represents
  A. conduction of the impulse throughout the atria.
  B. conduction of the impulse throughout the ventricles.
  C. ventricular repolarization.
  D. ventricular polarization.

LABELING ACTIVITY

Label the following heart positions.

Position of heart.

Label the structure indicated by the line; then match your answer with the label on the matching figure in chapter 16 of your textbook.

Label the following heart structures.

Blood low in oxygen

Blood high in oxygen

Heart chambers, valves, and circulation.

Label the structure indicated by the line; then match your answer with the label on the matching figure in chapter 16 of your textbook.

Label the following neck vessels.

Neck vessels.

Label the structure indicated by the line; then match your answer with the label on the matching figure in chapter 16 of your textbook.

■ Learner Activities

After reading Chapter 16, participate in the following learning activities.

WORKING WITH PEERS IN LEARNING LAB

1. Review the information in the Risk Factors box in Chapter 16. Determine your own risk for coronary heart disease (CHD). Identify ways to reduce your risk factors. Which ethnic groups are at higher risk for CHD?

2. Find an elderly client, friend, or relative whose heart and neck vessels you can examine. Discuss with your lab partner your assessment findings as they compare with those of a younger person.

3. Discuss with your lab partner what teaching would be appropriate to reduce an individual's risk for coronary heart disease (CHD).

INTERVIEWING AND RECORDING ASSESSMENT FINDINGS

Use the following Nursing History Checklist as your guide to interviewing and recording your findings in your heart and neck vessels assessment.

NURSING HISTORY CHECKLIST

Questions	Normal findings	Abnormal findings	Data missing
Current Symptoms			
1. Chest pain (type, location, radiation, duration, frequency, intensity)?			
2. Palpitations?			
3. Dizziness?			
4. Swollen ankles?			
Past History			
1. Previous heart problems: heart defect, murmur, heart attack (MI)?			
2. Previous diagnosis of rheumatic fever, hypertension, elevated cholesterol, diabetes mellitus?			
3. Heart surgery or cardiac balloon intervention?			
Family History			
1. Hypertension?			
2. Myocardial infarction?			
3. Coronary heart disease?			
4. Elevated cholesterol?			
5. Diabetes mellitus?			
Lifestyle and Health Practices			
1. Cigarette smoking pattern?			
2. Life stress-type and amount?			
3. Usual diet and exercise patterns?			
4. Use of alcohol?			
5. Sleep routine (use of extra pillows, up to urinate, feels rested)?			
6. Use of medications or treatments for heart disease?			
7. Self-monitoring of heart rate or blood pressure?			
8. Screenings for blood pressure, cholesterol, electrocardiogram (ECG)?			
9. Impact of CHD on sexual activity?			

PERFORMING PHYSICAL ASSESSMENT

Use the following Physical Assessment Checklist as your guide to performing a heart and neck vessel assessment.

PHYSICAL ASSESSMENT CHECKLIST

Assessment Skill	Findings (Normal or Abnormal) and Notes		Performance (Satisfactory, Needs Improvement, Unsatisfactory)		
	N	A	S	N	U
1. Gather equipment (stethoscope with bell diaphragm, small pillow, penlight or movable exam light, watch with second hand, two centimeter rulers).	☐	☐	☐	☐	☐
2. Explain procedure to client.	☐	☐	☐	☐	☐
3. Ask client to gown.	☐	☐	☐	☐	☐
Neck Vessels					
1. Auscultate carotid arteries for bruits.	☐	☐	☐	☐	☐
2. Palpate each carotid artery for amplitude and contour of the pulse, elasticity of the vessel, and thrills.	☐	☐	☐	☐	☐
3. Inspect for jugular venous pulse.	☐	☐	☐	☐	☐
4. Measure jugular venous pressure.	☐	☐	☐	☐	☐
Heart (Precordium)					
1. Inspect for visible pulsations (note if apical or other).	☐	☐	☐	☐	☐
2. Palpate apical pulse for location, size, strength, and duration of pulsation.	☐	☐	☐	☐	☐
3. Palpate for abnormal pulsations or vibrations at apex, left sternal border, and base.	☐	☐	☐	☐	☐
4. Auscultate heart sounds for rate and rhythm (apical and radial pulses, pulse rate deficit, S_1 and S_2).	☐	☐	☐	☐	☐
5. Auscultate S_1 and S_2 heart sounds for sound location and strength pattern (louder/softer at locations and with respiration, splitting of S_2).	☐	☐	☐	☐	☐
6. Auscultate for extra heart sounds (clicks, rubs) and murmurs (systolic or diastolic, intensity grade, pitch, quality, shape or pattern, location, transmission, effect of ventilation and position).	☐	☐	☐	☐	☐
7. Auscultate with the client in the left lateral position and with the client sitting up, leaning forward, and exhaling.	☐	☐	☐	☐	☐
Analysis of Data					
1. Formulate nursing diagnoses (wellness, risk, actual).	☐	☐	☐	☐	☐
2. Formulate collaborative problems.	☐	☐	☐	☐	☐
3. Make necessary referrals.	☐	☐	☐	☐	☐

CRITICAL THINKING AND CASE STUDIES

1. Your client states that his physician informed him that he has a new Grade 3 heart murmur. He asks you to explain the following to him in layman's terms:

   What is a heart murmur?

   What does grade 3 mean?

   What causes a heart murmur?

   What does my murmur sound like?

2. On the basis of the following assessment information, work through the steps of analyzing the data. Identify abnormal data and strengths in **subjective** and **objective findings**. Assemble **cue clusters**, draw **inferences**, make possible **nursing diagnoses**, identify **defining characteristics**, **confirm** or **rule out** the nursing diagnosis, and **document** your conclusions. Use the blank diagnostic analysis charts provided at the end of this book to guide your thinking. You may want to write on the chart or use separate paper. Propose nursing diagnoses that are specific to the client in the case study. Identify collaborative problems, if any, for this client. Finally, identify data, if any, that point toward a medical problem requiring a referral.

   Larry Manning is a 37-year-old African-American male client. He is a registered nurse and works 12-hour night shifts (7 p.m. to 7 a.m.) in an intensive care unit. He is married and has two daughters, aged 9 and 6. He has come to a local nurse practitioner for an annual physical examination. He is particularly worried about his risk for cardiac problems.

   When interviewed, Larry describes his general health as good. He denies any history of heart problems, surgery, or rheumatic fever and is not currently taking any medications. No previous lipid screening results are available. Larry states that he thinks his father has high blood pressure. He states that he drinks socially: one to two beers two to three times per week. He smokes about a half pack of cigarettes per day. He says, "I try to quit, but my job is so stressful, and smoking relaxes me." He states that he does not follow any specific diet, and he admits a weakness for sweets and chocolate. He denies any cough, dyspnea, chest pain, dizziness, palpitations, or swelling in his feet or legs. He states that he exercises sporadically, mainly playing tennis and basketball. He relates that he sometimes has difficulty sleeping during the day, and then uses that time to get some chores done.

   Physical examination reveals a blood pressure of 160/84 mm Hg. The carotid pulses are equal bilaterally, 2+, elastic; no bruits are auscultated. Jugular venous pulsation disappears when the client is upright. Jugular venous pressure is 2 cm. The precordium is intact, with uniform color and no visible pulsations, heaves, or lifts. The apical impulse palpated in the fifth intercostal space (ICS) at the left midclavicular line (MCL) and is approximately the size of a nickel, with no thrill. The apical heart rate is auscultated at 88 beats/minute, with regular rhythm; S_1 is heard best at the apex, S_2 is heard best at the base. No splitting, snaps, clicks, or murmurs are noted.

■ Chapter Post-test

MULTIPLE CHOICE QUESTIONS

Choose the one best answer for each of the following multiple-choice questions.

_____ 1. During a cardiac examination, the nurse can **best** hear the S1 heart sound by placing the stethoscope at the client's

    A. base of the heart.

    B. pulmonic valve area.

    C. apex of the heart.

    D. second left interspace.

_____ 2. The S4 heart sound

    A. can be heard during systole.

    B. is often termed *ventricular gallop*.

    C. is usually due to a heart murmur.

    D. can be heard during diastole.

_____ 3. An adult client visits the clinic and tells the nurse that she feels chest pain and pain down her left arm. The nurse should refer the client to a physician for possible

    A. congestive heart failure.

    B. angina.

    C. palpitations.

    D. acute anxiety reaction.

_____ 4. An adult client tells the nurse that his father died of a massive coronary at the age of 65. The nurse should explain to the client that one of the risk factors for coronary heart disease is

    A. high serum level of low-density lipoproteins.

    B. low carbohydrate diets.

    C. high serum level of high-density lipoproteins.

    D. diets that are high in antioxidant vitamins.

_____ 5. The nurse is planning a presentation about coronary heart disease for a group of middle-aged adults. Which of the following should be included in the nurse's teaching plan?

    A. Hispanic clients have a higher incidence of CHD than black or white Americans.

    B. The incidence of hypertension in the white population of the United States is greater than in the black population.

    C. Women are more likely to have serious stenosis after a heart attack.

    D. Estrogen replacement therapy in postmenopausal women decreases the risk of heart attack.

_____ 6. The nurse is preparing to assess the cardiovascular system of an adult client with emphysema. The nurse anticipates that there may be some difficulty palpating the client's

A. apical pulse.

B. breath sounds.

C. jugular veins.

D. carotid arteries.

_____ 7. The nurse is planning to auscultate a female adult client's carotid arteries. The nurse should plan to

A. ask the client to hold her breath.

B. palpate the arteries before auscultation.

C. place the diaphragm of the stethoscope over the artery.

D. ask the client to breathe normally.

_____ 8. While assessing an older adult client, the nurse detects a bruit over the carotid artery. The nurse should explain to the client that a bruit is

A. a normal sound heard in adult clients.

B. a wheezing sound.

C. associated with occlusive arterial disease.

D. heard when the artery is almost totally occluded.

_____ 9. The nurse assesses a hospitalized adult client and observes that the client's jugular veins are fully extended. The nurse contacts the client's physician because the client's signs are indicative of

A. pulmonary emphysema.

B. diastolic murmurs.

C. patent ductus arteriosus.

D. increased central venous pressure.

_____ 10. While palpating the apex, left sternal border, and base in an adult client, the nurse detects a thrill. The nurse should further assess the client for

A. cardiac murmur.

B. left-sided heart failure.

C. constrictive pericarditis.

D. congestive heart failure.

_____ 11. The nurse is auscultating the heart sounds of an adult client. To auscultate Erb's point, the nurse should place the stethoscope at the

A. second intercostal space at the right sternal border

B. third to fifth intercostal space at the left sternal border.

C. apex of the heart near the midclavicular line.

D. fourth or fifth intercostal space at the left lower sternal border.

_____ 12. While auscultating an adult client's heart rate and rhythm, the nurse detects a regular irregular pattern. The nurse should

A. assess the client for signs and symptoms of pulmonary disease.

B. document this as a normal finding.

C. schedule the client for an ECG.

D. refer the client to a physician.

_____ 13. The nurse has assessed the heart sounds of an adolescent client and detects the presence of an S3 heart sound at the beginning of the diastolic pause. The nurse should instruct the client that she should

    A. be referred to a cardiologist for further evaluation.

    B. be examined again in 6 months.

    C. restrict exercise and strenuous activities.

    D. recognize that this finding is normal in adolescents.

_____ 14. While assessing an adult client, the nurse detects opening snaps early in diastole during auscultation of the heart. The nurse should refer the client to a physician because this is usually indicative of

    A. pulmonary hypertension.

    B. aortic stenosis.

    C. mitral valve stenosis.

    D. pulmonary hypertension.

_____ 15. The nurse detects paradoxical pulses in an adult client during an examination. The nurse should explain to the client that paradoxical pulses are usually indicative of

    A. obstructive lung disease.

    B. left-sided heart failure.

    C. premature ventricular contractions.

    D. aortic stenosis.

_____ 16. The nurse is assessing an adult client with a diagnosis of sinus arrhythmia. The nurse should explain to the client that this indicates that the

    A. heartbeats are followed by a pause.

    B. ventricular contraction occurs irregularly.

    C. S1 and S2 sounds are both split.

    D. heart rate speeds up and slows down during a cycle.

_____ 17. The fourth heart sound, S4, is a/an

    A. low-frequency sound best heard with the bell of the stethoscope.

    B. abnormal finding in trained athletes.

    C. sound that can be heard in the absence of atrial contraction.

    D. sound that may increase during expiration.

CROSSWORD PUZZLE

Complete the following crossword puzzle to become more familiar with the terminology used with assessment of the neck vessels and heart.

ACROSS

1. Area of auscultation located at 2nd ICS at left sternal border
4. Part of stethoscope used to auscultate normal heart sounds
6. Localized area of tissue necrosis caused by prolonged anoxia
9. Assessment technique most often associated with evaluation of the cardiovascular system
10. Dorsalis _____: peripheral pulse located on dorsum of foot just lateral to tendon of great toe
11. Palpable murmur described as feeling like the throat of a purring cat
13. Abbreviation for specific area of the chest where the heartbeat is palpated most clearly

14. Area of auscultation located at the apex and assessing the left ventricle; 4th-5th ICS at lt. MCL
15. Peripheral pulse felt most often because of its accessibility
17. Event of the heart when contraction of the ventricles forces blood into major vessels
23. Area of auscultation at 2nd ICS and rt. sternal border
24. Palpable, diffuse, sustained lift of the chest wall or a portion of the wall
26. Audible variation between closure of two valves
27. An abnormally slowed heart rate, usually under 50 beats/minute

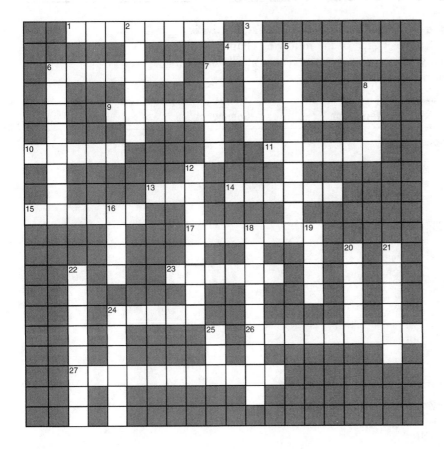

DOWN

2. Results of turbulent blood flow produced by pathologic condition of valvular or septal wall

3. Posterior _____; peripheral noted just behind the medial malleolus (ankle bone)

5. Classification of pulses detectable by feeling

6. Diminished blood supply to an organ or body part

7. Pressure waves that temporarily expand the wall of the artery from the propulsion of blood

8. The portion of the stethoscope used to assess for murmurs

12. Event in the heart cycle that involves relaxation of the ventricles

16. Most frequent location of S_3 and S_4 heart sounds; "point of the heart"

18. Area of auscultation located at the 4th-5th ICS at the left sternal border; evaluates rt. ventricle

19. "Point" located at the 3rd ICS at left sternal border: murmurs most often heard here

20. Audible murmur (a blowing sound heard in auscultating over a peripheral vessel or organ

21. Paroxysmal pain in chest, often associated with myocardial ischemia

22. Blood clot attached to the inner wall of a vessel; usually cause some degree of occlusion

24. Calf pain associated with rapid dorsiflexion of the foot: _____ sign

25. Abbreviation for the heart rate that originates within the SA node in right atrium

▪ Self-Reflection and Evaluation of Learner Objectives

After you have read Chapter 16 and completed the above quizzes and activities, please identify to what degree you have met each of the following chapter learning objectives. For those objectives that you have met partially or not at all, you will want to review chapter content for that learning objective.

Objective	Very much	Somewhat	Not at all
1. Describe the structure and functions of the heart and neck vessels.			
2. Describe the electrical conduction system of the heart.			
3. Describe each phase of the electrocardiogram (ECG).			
4. Discuss the two phases of the cardiac cycle.			
5. Describe normal heart sounds and extra heart sounds.			
6. Discuss possible conditions that contribute to extra heart sounds or heart murmurs.			
7. Discuss the components of the jugular venous pulse wave.			
8. Discuss risk factors for coronary heart disease (CHD) and ways to reduce these risk factors.			
9. Obtain an accurate nursing history of the client's heart and neck vessels.			
10. Prepare the client for an examination of the heart and neck vessels.			
11. Describe the equipment necessary to perform a heart and neck vessel assessment.			

Objective	Very much	Somewhat	Not at all
12. Describe the two physical examination techniques (auscultation and palpation) used to assess the neck vessels, and the three techniques (auscultation, palpation, and inspection) used to assess the precordium and heart sounds.			
13. Auscultate and palpate the carotid arteries for bruits, amplitude, regularity, and contour of the pulse, vessel elasticity, or presence of thrills. Inspect the jugular for visibility of pulse, and measure jugular venous pressure.			
14. Assess the heart and precordium for pulsations, heart sounds, heart rate, and rhythm.			
15. Identify appropriate nursing diagnoses and collaborative problems commonly seen with assessment of the heart and neck vessels.			

For additional information on this book, be sure to visit *http://connection.lww.com.*

Peripheral Vascular Assessment

CHAPTER OVERVIEW

The arteries and veins of the arms and legs, the lymphatic system, and the capillaries are the vessels of peripheral vascular circulation. They deliver and exchange blood and fluids to and from the arms, legs, hands, and feet. As such, their function is a key factor in mobility and health. Use the following exercises and quizzes to help you review and master basic techniques and skills for peripheral vascular assessment.

■ Chapter Pretest

Choose the one best answer for each of the following multiple-choice questions.

_____ 1. The major artery that supplies blood to the arm is the
   A. radial artery.
   B. ulnar artery.
   C. posterior artery.
   D. brachial artery.

_____ 2. The popliteal artery can be palpated at the
   A. knee.
   B. great toe.
   C. ankle.
   D. inguinal ligament.

_____ 3. The posterior tibial pulse can be palpated at the
   A. great toe.
   B. knee.
   C. top of the foot.
   D. ankle.

_____ 4. Blood from the lower trunk and legs drains upward into the inferior vena cava. The percentage of the body's blood volume that is contained in the veins is nearly
   A. 50%.
   B. 60%.
   C. 70%.
   D. 80%.

LABELING ACTIVITY

Label the following major arteries of the arms and legs.

Major arteries of the arms and legs.

Label the structure indicated by the line; then match your answer with the label on the matching figure in chapter 17 of your textbook.

Label the following major leg veins.

Major veins of the legs.

Label the structure indicated by the line; then match your answer with the label on the matching figure in chapter 17 of your textbook.

Label the following superficial lymph nodes of the arms and legs.

Superficial lymph nodes of the arms and legs.

Label the structure indicated by the line; then match your answer with the label on the matching figure in chapter 17 of your textbook.

■ Learner Activities

WORKING WITH PEERS IN LEARNING LAB

After reading Chapter 17, participate in the following learning activities.

1. Review the information in the Risk Factors display in Chapter 17. Determine your own risk for peripheral vascular disease. Identify ways to reduce your risk factors. Which ethnic groups are at higher risk for peripheral vascular disease?

2. Find an elderly client or friend or relative who will let you examine his or her peripheral vascular system. Discuss your assessment findings with your lab partner as they compare with those of a younger person.

3. Discuss with your lab partner what teaching would be appropriate to reduce an individual's risk of peripheral vascular disease.

INTERVIEWING AND RECORDING ASSESSMENT FINDINGS

Use the following Nursing History Checklist to interview a peer, friend, or family member regarding peripheral vascular status.

NURSING HISTORY CHECKLIST

Questions	Normal findings	Abnormal findings	Data missing
Current Symptoms			
1. Skin changes (color, temperature, or texture)?			
2. Leg pain, heaviness, or aching? Does it awaken you at night?			
3. Leg veins (rope-like, bulging, or contorted)?			
4. Leg sores or open wounds (location, pain)?			
5. Swelling in legs or feet?			
6. Men: Sexual activity changes?			
7. Swollen glands or nodules (pain)?			
Past History			
1. Previous problems with circulation in arms or legs (blood clots, ulcers, coldness, hair loss, numbness, swelling, or poor healing)?			
2. Heart or blood vessel surgeries or treatments (coronary artery bypass, repair of an aneurysm, or vein stripping)?			
Family History			
1. Family history of varicose veins, diabetes, hypertension, coronary heart disease, or elevated cholesterol or triglyceride levels?			
Lifestyle and Health Practices			
1. Cigarettes or other forms of tobacco, past or present use (explain: quantity and length of time)?			
2. Regular exercise?			
3. Women: use of oral contraceptives?			
4. Degree of stress?			
5. Peripheral vascular problems that interfere with ADLs?			
6. Use of medications to improve circulation or control blood pressure?			
7. Use of support hose?			

PERFORMING PHYSICAL ASSESSMENT

Use the following Physical Assessment Checklist as your guide to performing a peripheral vascular assessment.

PHYSICAL ASSESSMENT CHECKLIST

Assessment Skill	Findings (Normal or Abnormal) and Notes — N	A	Performance (Satisfactory, Needs Improvement, Unsatisfactory) — S	N	U
1. Gather equipment (gloves, centimeter tape, stethoscope, Doppler ultrasound probe, tourniquet).	☐	☐	☐	☐	☐
2. Explain procedure to client.	☐	☐	☐	☐	☐
3. Ask client to gown.	☐	☐	☐	☐	☐
Arms					
1. Inspect bilaterally for size, presence of edema, and venous patterning.	☐	☐	☐	☐	☐
2. Inspect bilaterally for skin color.	☐	☐	☐	☐	☐
3. Inspect fingertips for clubbing.	☐	☐	☐	☐	☐
4. Palpate fingers, hands, and arms for temperature, using dorsal surface of your fingers.	☐	☐	☐	☐	☐
5. Determine capillary refill time.	☐	☐	☐	☐	☐
6. Palpate radial, ulnar, and brachial pulses.	☐	☐	☐	☐	☐
7. Palpate for epitrochlear lymph nodes behind the elbow in the groove between the biceps and triceps muscles.	☐	☐	☐	☐	☐
8. Perform Allen's test by occluding the radial and ulnar arteries and observing for palm pallor. Then, release the ulnar artery and watch for color to return to hand.	☐	☐	☐	☐	☐
Legs					
1. Inspect bilaterally for skin color (client in supine position).	☐	☐	☐	☐	☐
2. Inspect bilaterally for distribution of hair.	☐	☐	☐	☐	☐
3. Inspect for lesions or ulcers (note whether margins are smooth and even, location such as at pressure points, size, depth, drainage, odor).	☐	☐	☐	☐	☐
4. Inspect for edema, unilateral or bilateral (if calves are asymmetrical, measure calf circumference).	☐	☐	☐	☐	☐
5. If client has edema, determine whether it is pitting or nonpitting. If client has pitting edema, rate on a 1+ to 4+ scale.	☐	☐	☐	☐	☐
6. Palpate skin temperature (cool, warm, hot). Use dorsal surface of hands.	☐	☐	☐	☐	☐
7. Palpate the superficial inguinal lymph nodes while keeping the genitals draped. If detected, note size, mobility, or tenderness.	☐	☐	☐	☐	☐
8. Palpate and auscultate femoral pulses over artery. Listen for bruits.	☐	☐	☐	☐	☐
9. Palpate popliteal, dorsalis pedis, and posterior tibial pulses.	☐	☐	☐	☐	☐
10. Inspect for varicosities and thrombophlebitis by asking client to stand.	☐	☐	☐	☐	☐

(continues)

PHYSICAL ASSESSMENT CHECKLIST (Continued)

Assessment Skill	Findings (Normal or Abnormal) and Notes		Performance (Satisfactory, Needs Improvement, Unsatisfactory)		
	N	A	S	N	U
11. Assess for arterial or venous insufficiency by—Eliciting bilaterally for Homans' sign by having client in supine position and	☐	☐	☐	☐	☐
a. flexing knee 5 degrees and quickly squeezing the muscle against the tibia	☐	☐	☐	☐	☐
OR					
b. with hand under slightly flexed knee, sharply dorsiflex the foot—Performing position change test for arterial insufficiency while client is in the supine position. Place hands under both of the client's ankles. Raise legs 12 inches above heart level, and ask client to pump feet up and down for 1 minute. Have client sit up and dangle legs. Note color of feet. Time the interval for color to return.	☐	☐	☐	☐	☐
12. If varicosities present, perform the manual compression test by having client stand. Firmly compress the lower portion of the varicose vein with one hand. Place other hand 6 to 8 inches above hand. Feel for pulsation in the upper hand.	☐	☐	☐	☐	☐
13. If varicosities are present, perform the Trendelenburg test with client in supine position. Elevate leg 90 degrees for 15 seconds. With legs elevated, apply a tourniquet to the upper thigh. Assist client to a standing position, and observe for venous filling. Remove tourniquet after 30 seconds, and watch for sudden filling of the varicose veins from above.	☐	☐	☐	☐	☐
Analysis of Data					
1. Formulate nursing diagnoses (wellness, risk, actual).	☐	☐	☐	☐	☐
2. Formulate collaborative problems.	☐	☐	☐	☐	☐
3. Make necessary referrals.	☐	☐	☐	☐	☐

■ Chapter Post-Test

MULTIPLE CHOICE

_____ 1. While assessing the peripheral vascular system of an adult client, the nurse detects cold, clammy skin and loss of hair on the client's legs. The nurse suspects that the client may be experiencing

A. venous stasis.

B. varicose veins.

C. thrombophlebitis.

D. arterial insufficiency.

_____ 2. During a physical examination, the nurse detects warm skin and brown pigmentation around an adult client's ankles. The nurse suspects that the client may be experiencing

A. venous insufficiency.

B. arterial occlusive disease.

C. venous ulcers.

D. ankle edema.

_____ 3. The nurse is assessing the peripheral vascular system of an older adult client. The client tells the nurse that her legs "seem cold all the time and sometimes feel tingly." The nurse suspects that the client may be experiencing

A. varicose veins.

B. intermittent claudication.

C. edema.

D. thrombophlebitis.

_____ 4. The nurse is caring for a client who is employed as a typist and has a family history of peripheral vascular disease. The nurse should instruct the client to reduce her risk factors by

A. eating a high-protein diet.

B. resting frequently.

C. drinking large quantities of milk.

D. getting regular exercise.

_____ 5. The nurse is preparing to use a Doppler ultrasound probe to detect blood flow in the femoral artery of an adult client. The nurse should

A. apply K-Y jelly to the client's skin.

B. place the client in a supine position with the head flat.

C. place the tip of the probe in a 30-degree angle to the artery.

D. apply gel used for electrocardiography (ECG) to the client's skin.

_____ 6. A client visits the clinic and tells the nurse that she had a mastectomy 2 years ago. The nurse should assess the client for

A. lymphedema.

B. Raynaud's disease.

C. poor peripheral pulses.

D. bruits over the radial artery.

_____ 7. After palpating the radial pulse of an adult client, the nurse suspects arterial insufficiency. The nurse should next assess the client's

A. femoral pulse.

B. popliteal pulse.

C. brachial pulse.

D. tibial pulse.

_____ 8. The nurse is preparing to palpate the epitrochlear lymph nodes of an adult male client. The nurse should instruct the client to

A. assume a supine position.

B. rest his arm on the examination table.

C. flex his elbow about 90 degrees.

D. make a fist with his left hand.

_____ 9. While inspecting the skin color of a male client's legs, the nurse observes that the client's legs are slightly cyanotic while he is sitting on the edge of the examination table. The nurse should refer the client to a physician for possible

A. arterial insufficiency.

B. congestive heart failure.

C. Raynaud's disease.

D. venous insufficiency.

_____ 10. While assessing the inguinal lymph nodes in an older adult client, the nurse detects that the lymph nodes are approximately 3 centimeters in diameter, nontender, and fixed. The nurse should refer the client to a physician because these findings are generally associated with

A. localized infection.

B. systemic infection.

C. arterial insufficiency.

D. malignancy.

_____ 11. The nurse plans to assess an adult client for Homans' sign. The nurse should

A. ask the client to remain standing for the procedure.

B. place the hands on the client's thigh muscle.

C. place the hands near the client's ankle.

D. flex the client's knee, then dorsiflex the foot.

_____ 12. The nurse is planning to perform the Trendelenburg test on an adult client. The nurse should explain to the client that this test is used to determine the

A. degree of arterial occlusion that exists.

B. pulse of a client with poor elasticity.

C. competence of the saphenous vein valves.

D. severity of thrombophlebitis.

MATCHING EXERCISE

Match the terms in the left column with the correct descriptions in the right column.

Term	Description
_____ 1. Doppler ultrasound probe	A. Deficient supply of oxygenated arterial blood to a tissue; caused by obstruction of a blood vessel
_____ 2. Edema	B. Swollen, distended, and knotted veins; occur most commonly in the legs
_____ 3. Clubbing	C. Usually occur on tips of toes, metatarsal heads, and lateral malleoli; ulcers have pale ischemic base, well-defined edges, and no bleeding
_____ 4. Raynaud's disease	
_____ 5. Capillary refill time	D. Swelling caused by excess fluid
_____ 6. Allen test	E. Usually occur on medial malleoli; ulcers have bleeding, uneven edges
_____ 7. Varicose veins	F. Calf pain elicited when the calf muscle is compressed against the tibia or when the foot is sharply dorsiflexed against the calf
_____ 8. Thrombophlebitis	
_____ 9. Homans' sign (positive)	G. The time it takes for color to return to the nailbeds after they have been blanched by pressure; a good measure of peripheral perfusion and cardiac output
_____ 10. Arterial ulcer	
_____ 11. Venous ulcer	H. Rigid peripheral blood vessels; occurs more commonly in older adults
_____ 12. Ischemia	I. Used to detect a weak peripheral pulse to monitor blood pressure in infants or children and to measure blood pressure in a lower extremity; It magnifies pulse sounds from the heart and blood vessels
_____ 13. Arteriosclerosis	
	J. Inflammation of a vein associated with thrombus formation
	K. Diffuse enlargement of terminal phalanges
	L. Determines the patency of the radial and ulnar arteries
	M. A vasospastic disorder, primarily affects the hands, characterized by color change from pallor, to cyanosis, to rubor; attacks precipitated by cold or emotional upset and relieved by warmth

ESSAY QUESTIONS

1. Explain how to differentiate between arterial and venous insufficiency.

2. Explain how to differentiate between edema associated with lymphedema versus edema associated with chronic venous insufficiency.

CRITICAL THINKING AND CASE STUDIES

1. On the basis of the following assessment information, work through the steps of analyzing the data. Identify abnormal data and strengths in **subjective** and **objective findings**. Assemble **cue clusters**, draw **inferences**, make possible **nursing diagnoses**, identify **defining characteristics**, **confirm** or **rule out** the nursing diagnosis, and **document** your conclusions. Use the blank diagnostic analysis charts provided at the end of this book to guide your thinking. You may want to write on the chart or use separate paper. Propose nursing diagnoses that are specific to the client in the case study. Identify collaborative problems, if any, for this client. Finally, identify data, if any, that point toward a medical problem requiring a referral.

Fran Hensley is an 84-year-old white widow with a medical diagnosis of venous (stasis) ulcers on the medial surface of her right lower leg. She is 4 feet 11 inches tall and weighs 100 pounds. She has been referred by her physician to the Visiting Nurse Association (VNA) for skilled visits three times a week by an R.N. She lives in a small rural community in her own home. She lives alone, but her older sister, aged 87 years, lives across the street and looks after her. Fran has one adult daughter, who is married and lives out of state.

When interviewed, Fran says she has had a history of venous ulcers for the past 10 years and has been seen in the past by the VNA for treatment of these ulcers. The last time she was seen for this was approximately 8 months ago, when she had venous ulcers on the medial aspects of both legs. Both areas were well healed at the time of discharge.

Although communication with Fran is difficult because of a hearing loss, she denies any pain from the ulcers. However, she does cry out at times during the dressing changes. Her sister provides most of the information for the nurses and states that Fran has been up more than usual during the past few weeks and does not rest with her legs elevated as much as she should. Fran can ambulate with the aid of a walker. Her sister checks on Fran several times during the day and prepares meals for her.

Physical assessment reveals the following findings on the upper extremities: no edema, pink, and no areas of discoloration observed bilaterally. The nailbeds have no signs of clubbing. The upper and lower arms are warm to touch; however, the hands are slightly cool to touch. Capillary refill time is normal. The radial and brachial pulses are strong bilaterally. The epitrochlear lymph nodes are nonpalpable. The ulnar pulses are nonpalpable. Results of Allen's test are normal.

Physical assessment of lower extremities reveals areas of brownish pigmentation at the ankles. The legs are warm to the touch. An area of ulceration approximately 4 centimeters × 7 centimeters is present on the medial aspect of the left ankle. The medial aspect of the right lower leg has an area of scar tissue approximately 3 centimeters × 8 centimeters. Both lower legs are thin, but the left leg is slightly swollen, with 1+ pitting edema. No varicosities are noted. The inguinal lymph nodes are nonpalpable, and the femoral pulses are strong and equal bilaterally. The popliteal pulses are absent, and the dorsalis pedal pulses are weak in both feet. The posterior tibial pulses are present but weak. Homans' sign is negative bilaterally. The client is unable to complete testing for arterial insufficiency.

■ Self-Reflection and Evaluation of Learner Objectives

After you have read Chapter 17 and completed the above review items, please identify to what degree you have met each of the following chapter learning objectives. For those objectives that you have met partially or not at all, you will want to review chapter content for that learning objective(s).

Objective	Very much	Somewhat	Not at all
1. Describe the structure and functions of the blood vessel walls.			
2. Describe capillary and lymphatic circulation.			
3. Discuss risk factors for peripheral vascular disease and ways to reduce these risk factors.			
4. Discuss the incidence of peripheral vascular disease across cultures.			
5. Obtain an accurate nursing history of the client's peripheral vascular system.			
6. Explain how to prepare the client for an examination of the peripheral vascular system.			
7. Describe the equipment necessary to perform an examination of the peripheral vascular system.			
8. Inspect the size, presence of edema, venous patterning, color, and clubbing of fingertips.			
9. Palpate the temperature of the client's fingers, hands, and arms.			
10. Assess the client's capillary refill time.			
11. Palpate the client's radial, ulnar, and brachial pulses.			
12. Assess the client for epitrochlear lymph nodes.			
13. Perform the Allen test on a client.			
14. Inspect and palpate the client's legs for color, hair distribution, lesions or ulcers, edema, and skin temperature.			
15. Palpate the client's inguinal area for the superficial inguinal lymph nodes.			
16. Palpate the client's femoral, popliteal, dorsalis pedis, and posterior tibial pulses.			
17. Inspect the client's legs for varicosities and thrombophlebitis.			
18. Assess the client for arterial and venous insufficiency of the legs.			

For additional information on this book, be sure to visit *http://connection.lww.com.*

Abdominal Assessment

CHAPTER OVERVIEW

The abdomen houses the structures of several different body systems—gastrointestinal, reproductive (female), lymphatic, and urinary. Known as the solid or hollow abdominal viscera, these structures include the liver, pancreas, spleen, adrenal glands, kidneys, ovaries, and uterus (solid viscera) and the stomach, gallbladder, small intestine, colon, and bladder (hollow viscera). Abdominal assessment is complex, largely because of the many vital organs and blood vessels within the abdominal cavity and the life-sustaining functions, such as digestion and elimination, that are performed there.

■ Chapter Pretest

MULTIPLE CHOICE

Choose the one best answer for each of the following multiple-choice questions.

_____ 1. The abdominal contents are enclosed externally by the abdominal wall musculature—three layers of muscle extending from the back, around the flanks, to the front. The outer muscle layer is the external

    A. rectal abdominis.

    B. transverse abdominis.

    C. abdominal oblique.

    D. umbilical oblique.

_____ 2. The sigmoid colon is located in this area of the abdomen: the

    A. left upper quadrant.

    B. left lower quadrant.

    C. right upper quadrant.

    D. right lower quadrant.

_____ 3. The pancreas of an adult client is located

    A. below the diaphragm and extending below the right costal margin.

    B. posterior to the left midaxillary line and posterior to the stomach.

    C. high and deep under the diaphragm, and can be palpated.

    D. deep in the upper abdomen, and is not normally palpable.

_____ 4. The primary function of the gallbladder is to

    A. store and excrete bile.

    B. aid in the digestion of protein.

C. produce alkaline mucus.

D. produce hormones.

_____ 5. The colon originates in this abdominal area: the

A. right lower quadrant.

B. right upper quadrant.

C. left lower quadrant.

D. left upper quadrant.

LABELING ACTIVITY

Label the landmarks of the abdomen in the following figure.

Landmarks of the abdomen.

Label the structure indicated by the line; then match your answer with the label on the matching figure in chapter 18 of your textbook.

Label the structures of the four quadrants and the nine regions of the abdomen in the following two figures.

Abdominal quadrants.

Label the structure indicated by the line; then match your answer with the label on the matching figure in chapter 18 of your textbook.

Label the organs of the abdomen in the following figure.

Abdominal viscera.

Label the structure indicated by the line; then match your answer with the label on the matching figure in chapter 18 of your textbook.

■ Learner Activities

After reading Chapter 18, participate in the following learning activities.

1. Practice preparing your lab partner for an abdominal exam. Discuss the purpose of emptying the bladder and positioning. Obtain the necessary equipment.

2. Review the Risk Factors box in Chapter 18. Then explain the abdominal skin changes that may be present in clients from various cultures.

3. Use a washable marker to mark off the four quadrants of the abdomen on your lab partner. Identify the organs found in each quadrant. Now have your partner mark with a washable marker the nine regions on your abdomen. Identify the organs found in each of the nine regions.

4. Inspect the skin and umbilicus of your lab partner. Discuss the differences between a deviated umbilicus and an everted umbilicus. Differentiate between abdominal respiratory movements, aortic pulsations, and peristaltic waves.

5. Measure the abdominal girth of your lab partner, and discuss the various causes of abdominal distention and asymmetry.

6. Auscultate bowel sounds; record their intensity, pitch, and frequency; and discuss the significance of bowel sounds, including the absence of bowel sounds. Also note where vascular sounds or friction rubs may occur and the significance of each.

7. Percuss the abdomen, and note the significance of the sounds heard.

8. Palpate the span of your partner's liver, documenting the size. Perform the scratch test.

9. Percuss your lab partner's spleen.

10. Perform light and deep palpation of your lab partner's abdomen.

11. Palpate your lab partner's liver and spleen. Discuss the significance of enlargement.

INTERVIEWING AND RECORDING ASSESSMENT FINDINGS

Use the following Nursing History Checklist as your guide to interviewing and recording findings in abdominal assessment.

NURSING HISTORY CHECKLIST

Questions	Normal findings	Abnormal findings	Data missing
Current Symptoms			
1. Abdominal pain present?			
2. What factors precipitate the pain or make it worse?			
3. Description and location of the pain?			
4. Other symptoms present, such as nausea, vomiting, diarrhea, appetite changes, constipation?			
5. Recent weight gain or loss?			
Past History			
1. Previous abdominal surgery/trauma/injury/medications?			
2. Previous abdominal pain and treatment?			
3. Results of any lab work or gastrointestinal studies?			
Family History			
1. Stomach, colon, or liver cancer?			
2. Abdominal pain, appendicitis, colitis, bleeding, or hemorrhoids?			
3. Person responsible for nutrition in family?			
Lifestyle and Health Practices			
1. Smoking, amount?			
2. Alcohol use, amount?			
3. Diet (food and drink), past 24 hours?			
4. Antacid use, amount?			
5. Medication use?			
6. Fluid intake?			
7. Exercise, amount?			
8. Cause of stress in life; effect on eating and elimination patterns?			
9. Past actions with abdominal pain or problems?			

PERFORMING PHYSICAL ASSESSMENT

Use the following Physical Assessment Checklist as your guide to performing an abdominal assessment.

PHYSICAL ASSESSMENT CHECKLIST

Assessment Skill	Findings (Normal or Abnormal) and Notes		Performance (Satisfactory, Needs Improvement, Unsatisfactory)		
	N	A	S	N	U
1 Gather equipment (pillow/towel, centimeter ruler, stethoscope, marking pen).	☐	☐	☐	☐	☐
2. Explain procedure to client.	☐	☐	☐	☐	☐
3. Ask client to gown.	☐	☐	☐	☐	☐
Abdomen					
1. Inspect the skin, noting color, vascularity, striae, scars, and lesions (wear gloves to inspect lesions).	☐	☐	☐	☐	☐
2. Inspect the umbilicus, noting color, location, and contour.	☐	☐	☐	☐	☐
3. Inspect the contour of the abdomen.	☐	☐	☐	☐	☐
4. Inspect the symmetry of the abdomen.	☐	☐	☐	☐	☐
5. Inspect abdominal movement, noting respiratory movement, aortic pulsations, and/or peristaltic waves.	☐	☐	☐	☐	☐
6. Auscultate for bowel sounds, noting intensity, pitch, and frequency.	☐	☐	☐	☐	☐
7. Auscultate for vascular sounds and friction rubs.	☐	☐	☐	☐	☐
8. Percuss the abdomen for tone.	☐	☐	☐	☐	☐
9. Percuss the liver.	☐	☐	☐	☐	☐
10. Perform the scratch test.	☐	☐	☐	☐	☐
11. Percuss the spleen.	☐	☐	☐	☐	☐
12. Perform blunt percussion on the liver and the kidneys.	☐	☐	☐	☐	☐
13. Perform light palpation, noting tenderness or guarding in all quadrants.	☐	☐	☐	☐	☐
14. Perform deep palpation, noting tenderness or masses in all quadrants.	☐	☐	☐	☐	☐
15. Palpate the umbilicus.	☐	☐	☐	☐	☐
16. Palpate the aorta.	☐	☐	☐	☐	☐
17. Palpate the liver, noting consistency and tenderness.	☐	☐	☐	☐	☐
18. Palpate the spleen, noting consistency and tenderness.	☐	☐	☐	☐	☐
19. Palpate the kidneys.	☐	☐	☐	☐	☐
20. Palpate the urinary bladder.	☐	☐	☐	☐	☐
21. Perform the test for shifting dullness.	☐	☐	☐	☐	☐
22. Perform the fluid wave test.	☐	☐	☐	☐	☐
23. Perform the ballottement test.	☐	☐	☐	☐	☐
24. Perform tests for appendicitis:	☐	☐	☐	☐	☐
rebound tenderness	☐	☐	☐	☐	☐

(continues)

PHYSICAL ASSESSMENT CHECKLIST *(Continued)*

Assessment Skill	Findings (Normal or Abnormal) and Notes		Performance (Satisfactory, Needs Improvement, Unsatisfactory)		
	N	A	S	N	U
Rovsing's sign	☐	☐	☐	☐	☐
referred rebound tenderness	☐	☐	☐	☐	☐
psoas sign	☐	☐	☐	☐	☐
obturator sign	☐	☐	☐	☐	☐
hypersensitivity test	☐	☐	☐	☐	☐
25. Perform test for cholecystitis (Murphy's sign).	☐	☐	☐	☐	☐
Analysis of Data					
1. Formulate nursing diagnoses (wellness, risk, actual).	☐	☐	☐	☐	☐
2. Formulate collaborative problems.	☐	☐	☐	☐	☐
3. Make necessary referrals.	☐	☐	☐	☐	☐

■ Chapter Post-test

Choose the one best answer for each of the following multiple-choice questions.

_____ 1. To percuss the liver of an adult client, the nurse should begin the abdominal assessment at the client's

    A. right upper quadrant.

    B. right lower quadrant.

    C. left upper quadrant.

    D. left lower quadrant.

_____ 2. To palpate for tenderness of an adult client's appendix, the nurse should begin the abdominal assessment at the client's

    A. left upper quadrant

    B. left lower quadrant.

    C. right upper quadrant.

    D. right lower quadrant.

_____ 3. To palpate the spleen of an adult client, the nurse should begin the abdominal assessment of the client at the

    A. left lower quadrant

    B. left upper quadrant.

    C. right upper quadrant.

    D. right lower quadrant.

_____ 4. The nurse plans to assess an adult client's kidneys for tenderness. The nurse should assess the area at the

    A. right upper quadrant

    B. left upper quadrant.

C. external oblique angle.

D. costovertebral angle.

_____ 5. A client visits the clinic because she experienced bright hematemesis yesterday. The nurse should refer the client to a physician because this symptom is indicative of

A. stomach ulcers.

B. pancreatic cancer.

C. decreased gastric motility.

D. abdominal tumors.

_____ 6. The nurse is assessing an older adult client who has lost 5 pounds since her last visit 1 year ago. The client tells the nurse that her husband died 2 months ago. The nurse should further assess the client for

A. peptic ulcer.

B. bulimia.

C. appetite changes.

D. pancreatic disorders.

_____ 7. A client visits the clinic for a routine examination. The client tells the nurse she has become constipated because she is taking iron tablets prescribed for anemia. The nurse has instructed the client about the use of iron preparations and possible constipation. The nurse determines that the client has understood the instructions when she says

A. "I can decrease the constipation if I eat foods high in fiber and drink water."

B. "I should cut down on the number of iron tablets I am taking each day."

C. "Constipation should decrease if I take the iron tablets with milk."

D. "I should discontinue the iron tablets and eat foods that are high in iron."

_____ 8. The nurse is caring for a female client during her first postoperative day after a temporary colostomy. The client refuses to look at the colostomy bag or the area. A priority nursing diagnosis for this client is

A. denial related to temporary colostomy.

B. fear related to potential outcome of surgery.

C. disturbed body image related to temporary colostomy.

D. altered role functioning related to frequent colostomy bag changes.

_____ 9. The nurse is preparing to assess the abdomen of a hospitalized client 2 days after abdominal surgery. The nurse should first

A. palpate the incision site.

B. auscultate for bowel sounds.

C. percuss for tympany.

D. inspect the abdominal area.

_____ 10. The nurse is planning to assess the abdomen of an adult male client. Before the nurse begins the assessment, the nurse should

    A. ask the client to empty his bladder.

    B. place the client in a side-lying position.

    C. ask the client to hold his breath for a few seconds.

    D. tell the client to raise his arms above his head.

_____ 11. The nurse is assessing the abdomen of an adult client and observes a purple discoloration at the flanks. The nurse should refer the client to a physician for possible

    A. liver disease.

    B. abdominal distention.

    C. Cushing's syndrome.

    D. internal bleeding.

_____ 12. While assessing an adult client's abdomen, the nurse observes that the client's umbilicus is deviated to the left. The nurse should refer the client to a physician for possible

    A. gallbladder disease.

    B. cachexia.

    C. kidney trauma.

    D. masses.

_____ 13. While assessing an adult client's abdomen, the nurse observes that the client's umbilicus is enlarged and everted. The nurse should refer the client to a physician for possible

    A. umbilical hernia.

    B. ascites.

    C. intra-abdominal bleeding.

    D. pancreatitis.

_____ 14. The nurse assesses an adult male client's abdomen and observes diminished abdominal respiration. The nurse determines that the client should be further assessed for

    A. liver disease.

    B. umbilical hernia.

    C. intestinal obstruction.

    D. peritoneal irritation.

_____ 15. The nurse is assessing the bowel sounds of an adult client. After listening to each quadrant, the nurse determines that bowel sounds are not present. The nurse should refer the client to a physician for possible

    A. aortic aneurysm.

    B. paralytic ileus.

    C. gastroenteritis.

    D. fluid and electrolyte imbalances.

_____ 16. While assessing the abdominal sounds of an adult client, the nurse hears high-pitched, tingling sounds throughout the distended abdomen. The nurse should refer the client to a physician for possible

A. intestinal obstruction.

B. gastroenteritis.

C. inflamed appendix.

D. cirrhosis of the liver.

_____ 17. During a physical examination of an adult client, the nurse is preparing to auscultate the client's abdomen. The nurse should

A. palpate the abdomen before auscultation.

B. listen in each quadrant for 15 seconds.

C. use the diaphragm of the stethoscope.

D. begin auscultation in the left upper quadrant.

_____ 18. To palpate the spleen of an adult client, the nurse should

A. ask the client to exhale deeply.

B. place the right hand below the left costal margin.

C. point the fingers of the left hand downward.

D. ask the client to remain in a supine position.

_____ 19. The nurse is planning to assess a client's abdomen for rebound tenderness. The nurse should

A. perform this abdominal assessment first.

B. ask the client to assume a side-lying position.

C. palpate lightly while slowly releasing pressure.

D. palpate deeply while quickly releasing pressure.

_____ 20. To assess an adult client for possible appendicitis and a positive psoas sign, the nurse should

A. rotate the client's knee internally.

B. palpate at the lower right quadrant.

C. raise the client's right leg from the hip.

D. support the client's right knee and ankle.

CRITICAL THINKING AND CASE STUDIES

1. Suppose you find that a client's abdomen is distended, pale, and taut. Describe the tests you might perform, differentiating between the fluid wave test and the test for shifting dullness.

2. You suspect that a client may have appendicitis. Identify and describe a variety of tests that can be used to detect appendicitis.

3. You suspect that a client may have cholecystitis. Identify and describe the test used to detect cholecystitis.

4. Janet Smith is 63 years old. She has a diagnosis of rheumatoid arthritis, for which she takes 8 to 10 aspirins daily to relieve pain. She states that for the past couple of days her stools have been dark and tarry-looking, and her stomach has been upset and "queasy." Hoping to settle her stomach, she changed her diet in the past 2 days to include only soups and fluids. She tells you that the only other medication she takes is a calcium supplement.

a. Describe the most likely cause for the client's upset stomach.

b. Describe the type of precipitating factors you would expect to find during an interview with Ms. Smith.

5. On the basis of the following assessment information, work through the steps of analyzing the data. Identify abnormal data and strengths in **subjective and objective findings**, assemble **cue clusters**, draw **inferences**, make possible **nursing diagnoses**, identify **defining characteristics, confirm or rule out** the nursing diagnosis, and **document** your conclusions.

Use the blank diagnostic analysis charts provided at the end of this book to guide your thinking. You may want to write on the chart or use separate paper. Propose nursing diagnoses that are specific to the client in the case study. Identify collaborative problems, if any, for this client. Finally, identify data, if any, that point toward a medical problem requiring a referral

Mrs. Vera Wagner is a 60-year-old white woman who emigrated from Germany to the United States at the age of 18. She has come to her primary care physician's office with her daughter. She tells you, "My daughter made me come here because I have had bad stomach pains for about 6 weeks." After you ask about the character, onset, location, duration, severity, and pattern of the pain as well as associated symptoms (COLDSPA), such as what relieves the pain and what functions are affected by pain, you learn the following information. The pain is aching epigastric pain, fairly continuous, and worse at night. It radiates to her back when she lies down. The pain gets progressively worse, is not affected by eating, and interferes with her daily function (it prevented her from attending her grandson's birthday party; it also wakes her up at night). Additionally, Mrs. Wagner admits to loss of appetite, mild nausea, heartburn, and fatigue. For the past several months she has felt full soon after beginning a meal. She tells you that she was afraid to tell her doctor this because "He always says I worry too much."

A review of Mrs. Wagner's chart discloses that she had four normal vaginal deliveries, several bladder and kidney infections, a total abdominal hysterectomy at age 50 for uterine fibroids, cholecystectomy at age 55, two episodes of deep vein thrombosis in the past few years, allergy to penicillin, and stomach sensitivity to medicines (e.g., aspirin). Four years ago she had gastric endoscopy and upper gastrointestinal (GI) barium swallow studies for complaints of heartburn and difficulty swallowing. The results revealed delayed esophageal peristalsis.

Mrs. Wagner takes estrogen and calcium daily (in the form of Tums) as recommended by her physician as a source of hormone and calcium after surgical menopause. She tells you that she has recently started to take acetaminophen once—sometimes twice—daily in the hope that this will relieve her pain. She has had mild temporary relief as a result.

Mrs. Wagner's family history reveals that her mother died at age 58 from "liver problems after having half her stomach removed." Mrs. Wagner says she does not smoke, drink, or use drugs. She says that she has eaten the same diet all her life. "I eat good German food, a lot of potatoes and meats. My children tell me I should eat more vegetables and drink more water, but I don't like fruits and vegetables and I'd rather drink coffee." In response to your question about exercise, you learn that Mrs. Wagner walks to the post office every day, and "I pick up after my husband around the house–does that count?" You comment that Mrs. Wagner looks upset, and she tells you that she is very concerned about her pain. "I have always been strong and healthy, and now I am getting old and sick. It is depressing."

Your physical assessment reveals a firmly palpable left supraclavicular node, approximately 2 centimeters in diameter, nonmobile, and nontender, as well as the following abdominal findings: abdomen round and symmetric, hysterectomy scar, striae, umbilicus in the midline without inflammation or herniation, slight midline pulsation in the epigastrium. Soft bowel sounds are heard in all four quadrants; no audible bruits. Generalized tympany percussed throughout; span of liver dullness is 13 centimeters over the midclavicular line (MCL), splenic dullness at the 10th intercostal space (ICS), MAL. The abdomen soft and tender to palpation in the epigastrium; the liver edge descends 2 centimeters below the right costal margin (RCM) on deep inspiration; no splenomegaly is noted.

■ Self-Reflection and Evaluation of Learner Objectives

After you have read Chapter 18 and completed the above review items, please identify to what extent you have met each of the following chapter learning objectives. For those you have met partially or not at all, you will want to review chapter content for that learning objective.

Objective	Very much	Somewhat	Not at all
1. Describe the structures and the functions of the abdomen.			
2. Identify the organs located in each of the quadrants and the nine regions of the abdomen.			
3. Obtain an accurate nursing history of the client's abdomen and functions.			
4. Differentiate between the three major types of abdominal pain.			
5. Describe how to prepare a client for an abdominal exam, and identify the equipment needed.			
6. Auscultate the abdomen for bowel sounds, vascular sounds, and friction rubs.			
7. Percuss the quadrants of the abdomen, noting the underlying structures, and liver and spleen spans.			
8. Perform light and deep palpation of the abdomen, noting any abnormalities.			
9. Describe the tests for ballottement and shifting dullness.			
10. Describe the five different tests used to detect appendicitis.			
11. Describe the test used to detect cholecystitis.			

For additional information on this book, be sure to visit *http://connection.lww.com.*

CHAPTER 19

Male Genitalia Assessment

CHAPTER OVERVIEW

An assessment of male genital structures requires an understanding of both the external and the internal genitalia as well as the inguinal (or groin) structures, because hernias are common in this area. Throughout the assessment, the nurse should keep in mind that Western culture emphasizes the importance of the male sex role and that self-esteem and body image are entwined with the male sex role. Therefore, the assessment may be uncomfortable or embarrassing for the client as well as the nurse. The key goals of the assessment are screening and detection of serious or life-threatening problems, such as testicular cancer, and patient education and health promotion. Use the following exercises and quizzes to help you review basic techniques and skills.

■ Chapter Pretest

Choose the one best answer for each of the following multiple-choice questions.

_____ 1. The corpora spongiosum extends distally to form the acorn-shaped
   A. glans.
   B. frenulum.
   C. corona.
   D. scrotum.

_____ 2. If a male client is uncircumcised, the glans of the penis is covered by the
   A. epididymis.
   B. frenulum.
   C. corona.
   D. foreskin.

_____ 3. The testes in the male scrotum are
   A. joined with the ejaculatory duct.
   B. suspended by the spermatic cord.
   C. able to produce progesterone.
   D. the location of the vas deferens.

_____ 4. The inguinal canal in a male client is located
   A. just above and parallel to the inguinal ligament.
   B. anteriorly above the symphysis pubis.
   C. anterior to the external inguinal ring.
   D. posterior to the superior iliac ring.

■ Labeling Activity

Label the following structures of the external and internal genitalia.

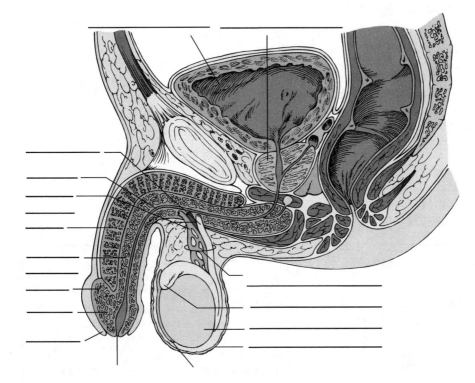

External and internal genitalia.

Label the structure indicated by the line; then match your answer with the label on the matching figure in chapter 19 of your textbook.

Label the following structures of the inguinal area.

Inguinal area.

Label the structure indicated by the line; then match your answer with the label on the matching figure in chapter 19 of your textbook.

■ Learner Activities

After reading Chapter 19, participate in the following learning activities.

WORKING WITH PEERS IN THE LEARNING LAB

1. Review the information in the Risk Factors box in Chapter 19 of the textbook. Determine your own risk for HIV/AIDS. Identify ways to reduce your risk factors. Which groups are at higher risk for contracting HIV/AIDS?

2. Obtain brochures and literature on sexually transmitted diseases (STDs) from the county health department or your campus student health center. Discuss with your lab partner the best way to give a presentation on this topic to teenagers and then to a college-aged group.

3. Obtain information from the American Cancer Society, the county health department, or your campus student health center on testicular cancer and testicular self-examination. Review the material with a lab partner, and discuss how you would teach a client how to examine himself.

DISPLAY 19-1. TESTICULAR SELF-EXAMINATION (TSE)

Testicular self-examination (TSE) is to be performed once a month; it is neither difficult nor time consuming. A convenient time is often after a warm bath or shower when the scrotum is more relaxed.

1. Use both hands to palpate the testis; the normal testicle is smooth and uniform in consistency.

2. With the index and middle fingers under the testis and the thumb on top, roll the testis gently in a horizontal plane between the thumb and fingers (A).

3. Feel for any evidence of a small lump or abnormality.

4. Follow the same procedure and palpate upward along the testis (B).

5. Locate the epididymis (C), a cordlike structure on the top and back of the testicle that stores and transports sperm.

6. Repeat the examination for the other testis. It is normal to find that one testis is larger than the other.

7. If you find any evidence of a small, pealike lump, consult your physician. It may be due to an infection or a tumor growth.

---

4. Using a model of the male genitalia, review the anatomy and function of each anatomic structure. Discuss the assessment findings with your lab partner, then compare those findings with what you would find in an elderly man.

INTERVIEWING AND RECORDING ASSESSMENT FINDINGS

Because of the sensitive nature of completing a male genitalia assessment, you will want to conduct a nursing history either by using a case study provided by your instructor or by having your lab partner assume the role of a fictitious client to answer the questions. Use the following Nursing History Checklist for your interview.

NURSING HISTORY CHECKLIST

Questions	Normal findings	Abnormal findings	Data missing
Current Symptoms			
1. Pain in penis, scrotum, testes, or groin?			
2. Lesions on penis or genital area?			
3. Lumps, swelling, or masses in scrotum, genital, or groin area?			
4. Heaviness or dragging feeling in scrotum?			
5. Difficulty urinating (hesitancy, frequency, or difficulty starting or maintaining a stream)?			
6. Changes in color, odor, or amount of urine?			
7. Pain or burning when urinating?			
8. Incontinence or dribbling of urine?			
9. Recent changes in sexual activity pattern or sexual desire?			
10. Difficulty attaining or maintaining an erection? Problems with ejaculation?			
11. Fertility problems?			
Past History			
1. Previous problems related to your pelvic area (surgeries, treatments, and results)?			
2. Date of last testicular exam by physician or nurse practitioner? Results?			
3. Tested for HIV? Why tested? Results?			
Family History			
1. Family history of prostate or testicular cancer? What type, and which family member(s)?			
Lifestyle and Health Practices			
1. Number of sexual partners?			
2. Kind of birth control method?			
3. Current or past exposure to chemicals or radiation?			

(continues)

NURSING HISTORY CHECKLIST (Continued)

Questions	Normal findings	Abnormal findings	Data missing
4. Usual daily activity?			
5. Heavy lifting?			
6. Genital problems that affect daily activities?			
7. Fertility concerns? Effect on relationship?			
8. Sexual preference?			
9. Concerns related to sex?			
10. Stress related to sex?			
11. Knowledge of sexually transmitted diseases and prevention?			
12. Do you perform testicular self-examination? Date last performed?			

PERFORMING PHYSICAL ASSESSMENT

Use the following Physical Assessment Checklist as your guide to performing an assessment of male genitalia.

PHYSICAL ASSESSMENT CHECKLIST

Assessment Skill	Findings (Normal or Abnormal) and Notes		Performance (Satisfactory, Needs Improvement, Unsatisfactory)		
	N	A	S	N	U
1. Gather equipment (gloves, stool, gown, penlight).	☐	☐	☐	☐	☐
2. Explain procedure to client.	☐	☐	☐	☐	☐
3. Ask client to put on gown.	☐	☐	☐	☐	☐
Penis					
1. Inspect the base of penis and pubic hair for growth pattern and excoriation, erythema, or infestation (client is standing while you sit).	☐	☐	☐	☐	☐
2. Inspect the skin of the shaft for rashes, lesions, or lumps.	☐	☐	☐	☐	☐
3. Palpate the shaft for hardened areas or areas of tenderness.	☐	☐	☐	☐	☐
4. Inspect the foreskin (if present) for color, location, and integrity.	☐	☐	☐	☐	☐
5. Inspect the glans for size, shape, lesions or redness, and location of the urinary meatus on the glans (if uncircumcised, ask him to retract his foreskin to allow for observation).	☐	☐	☐	☐	☐
6. Palpate for urethral discharge by gently squeezing the glans between the index finger and thumb.	☐	☐	☐	☐	☐
Scrotum					
1. Inspect the size, shape, and position (penis is held out of the way).	☐	☐	☐	☐	☐
2. Observe for swelling, lumps, or bulges.	☐	☐	☐	☐	☐
3. Inspect the skin for color, integrity, and the presence of lesions or rashes. (Spread out the scrotal folds of skin to perform an accurate inspection. Lift the sac to inspect the posterior skin.)	☐	☐	☐	☐	☐

PHYSICAL ASSESSMENT CHECKLIST

Assessment Skill	Findings (Normal or Abnormal) and Notes		Performance (Satisfactory, Needs Improvement, Unsatisfactory)		
	N	A	S	N	U
4. Palpate the scrotal contents (testes and epididymis) between your thumb and first two fingers. Note size, shape, consistency, and presence of tenderness or nodules. Palpate each spermatic cord and vas deferens, noting nodules, swelling, or tenderness.	☐	☐	☐	☐	☐
	☐	☐	☐	☐	☐
5. Transilluminate the scrotal contents (if a mass or swelling was noted). Look for a red glow.	☐	☐	☐	☐	☐

Inguinal Area

	N	A	S	N	U
1. Inspect for inguinal and femoral hernia, watching for bulges while the client bears down.	☐	☐	☐	☐	☐
2. Palpate for inguinal hernia, observing for bulges or masses. Have client shift weight to the left to palpate the right inguinal canal. Place index finger into the right scrotum, and press upward to the slit-like opening of the external inguinal ring. With finger in canal or external inguinal ring, ask him to bear down or cough. Repeat for left side.	☐	☐	☐	☐	☐
3. Palpate for femoral hernia on the front of the thigh in the femoral canal area. Ask him to bear down or cough while feeling for bulges. Repeat on the other side.	☐	☐	☐	☐	☐
4. Inspect and palpate for scrotal hernia (if a mass was detected during inspection or palpation of the scrotum). Ask client to lie down, and note whether the bulge disappears. If it remains, auscultate it for bowel sounds. Then, gently palpate the mass, and try to push it up into the abdomen unless it is too tender.	☐	☐	☐	☐	☐

Analysis of Data

	N	A	S	N	U
1. Formulate nursing diagnoses (wellness, risk, actual).	☐	☐	☐	☐	☐
2. Formulate collaborative problems.	☐	☐	☐	☐	☐
3. Make necessary referrals	☐	☐	☐	☐	☐

■ Chapter Post-test

_____ 1. During assessment of an elderly male client, the client tells the nurse that he has had difficulty urinating for the past few weeks. The nurse should refer the client to the physician for possible

A. inguinal hernia.

B. sexually transmitted disease.

C. impotence.

D. prostate enlargement.

_____ 2. A 25-year-old client asks the nurse how often he should have a testicular examination. After instructing the client about the American Cancer Society's guidelines, the nurse determines that the client has understood the instructions when he says he should have a testicular examination every

A. year.

B. 2 years.

C. 3 years.

D. 4 years.

_____ 3. A 45-year-old male client tells the nurse that he has had problems in having an erection for the last couple of weeks but is "doing better now." The nurse should explain to the client that

A. transient periods of erectile dysfunction are common.

B. impotence in males should be investigated.

C. transient impotence may be indicative of prostate enlargement.

D. inguinal hernias have been associated with transient impotence.

_____ 4. A male client tells the nurse that his occupation requires heavy lifting and a great deal of strenuous activity. The nurse should assess the client for

A. signs and symptoms of prostate enlargement.

B. erectile dysfunction.

C. inguinal hernia.

D. urinary tract infection.

_____ 5. During assessment of an adult client, which of the following lifestyle practices would indicate to the nurse that the client may be at high risk for HIV/AIDS? A client who

A. uses a condom on a regular basis.

B. has multiple female partners.

C. smokes marijuana occasionally.

D. has anal intercourse with other males.

_____ 6. During assessment of the genitalia of an adult male, the client has an erection. The nurse should

A. explain to the client that this often happens during an examination.

B. cover the client's genitals and discontinue the examination.

C. allow the client time to rest before proceeding with the examination.

D. continue the examination in an unhurried manner.

_____ 7. Before beginning the examination of the genitalia of an adult male client, the nurse should

A. ask the client to empty his bladder.

B. tell the client that he will remain in a supine position.

C. ask the client to leave his shirt in place.

D. tell the client that he may leave his underwear in place.

_____ 8. While assessing an adult male client, the nurse detects pimple-like lesions on the client's glans. The nurse explains the need for a referral to the client. The nurse determines that the client has understood the instructions when the client says he may have

    A. venereal warts.

    B. herpes infection.

    C. syphilis.

    D. gonorrhea.

_____ 9. While inspecting the genitalia of a male client, the nurse observes a chancre lesion under the foreskin. The nurse has explained this observation to the client. The nurse determines that the client understands the need for a referral when the client says that chancre lesions are associated with

    A. herpesvirus.

    B. syphilis

    C. papillomavirus.

    D. gonorrhea.

_____ 10. A male client visits the clinic and tells the nurse that he has had a white discharge from his penis for the past few days. The nurse should refer the client to a physician for possible

    A. urethritis.

    B. gonorrhea.

    C. herpes infection.

    D. syphilis.

_____ 11. The nurse has assessed a male client and determines that one of the testes is absent. The nurse should explain to the client that this condition is termed

    A. hypospadias.

    B. hematocele.

    C. cryptorchidism.

    D. orchitis.

_____ 12. The nurse is assessing the genitalia of an adult male client when he tells the nurse that his testes are swollen and painful. The nurse should refer the client to a physician for possible

    A. cancer.

    B. hydrocele.

    C. epididymitis.

    D. hematocele.

_____ 13. While transilluminating the scrotal contents in a male adult client, the nurse does not detect a red glow. The nurse should refer the client to a physician for possible

    A. spermatocele.

    B. orchitis.

    C. hydrocele.

    D. varicocele.

_____ 14. The nurse suspects that a male client may have a hernia. The nurse should further assess the client for

    A. bruising at the site.

    B. urinary tract infection.

    C. cysts at the spermatic cord.

    D. bowel sounds at the bulge.

_____ 15. A male client tells the nurse that he has received a diagnosis of hernia. He visits the clinic because he is nauseated and has extreme tenderness on the left side. The nurse should

    A. refer the client to an emergency room.

    B. try to push the mass into the abdomen.

    C. assess for a mass on the right side.

    D. assess the client's vital signs.

MATCHING

Match the terms in the left column with the correct descriptions in the right column.

Term	Description
_____ 1. Corona	A. Retracted foreskin that cannot be returned to cover the glans
_____ 2. Hernia	B. Displacement of the urinary meatus to the dorsal surface of the penis
_____ 3. Chancres	C. Base of the glans
_____ 4. Phimosis	D. Undescended testicle
_____ 5. Paraphimosis	E. Protrusion of bowel through weakened muscles
_____ 6. Hypospadias	F. A tight foreskin that cannot be retracted
_____ 7. Epispadias	G. Red, oval ulcerations caused by syphilis
_____ 8. Cryptorchidism	H. Displacement of the urinary meatus to the ventral surface of the penis

CRITICAL THINKING AND CASE STUDIES

1. Why would it be necessary to transilluminate the scrotal contents, and what are the possible findings and their significance?

2. During assessment for a hernia, what is the rationale for asking the client to cough or bear down?

3. Compare and contrast how you would focus the nursing history of the male genitalia for an 18-year-old versus that for an 80-year-old.

4. On the basis of the following assessment information, work through the steps of analyzing the data. Identify abnormal data and strengths in **subjective and objective findings,** assemble **cue clusters,** draw **inferences,** make possible **nursing diagnoses,** identify **defining characteristics, confirm or rule out** the nursing diagnosis, and **document** your conclusions.

    Use the blank diagnostic analysis charts provided at the end of this book to guide your thinking. You may want to write on the chart or use separate paper. Propose nursing diagnoses that are specific to the client in the case study.

Identify collaborative problems, if any, for this client. Finally, identify data, if any, that point toward a medical problem requiring a referral.

Don Carse is a 32-year-old African-American man who arrives at the clinic for an evaluation by a nurse practitioner. He complains that his right testicle feels heavy or weighted down. He appears very nervous and explains that he has been experiencing this feeling for about 3 months. He explains that he came in today because "my wife is very upset about it and pleaded with me to go to a doctor." When interviewed, the client reports that he doesn't have trouble becoming erect, but he states, "I feel like it takes longer to ejaculate." He denies past medical problems or a family history of cancer.

He explains that he hasn't had a genital examination in years—"I really don't like to go to the doctor unless I have a problem." He says he has never done, and does not really know how to do, a testicular self-examination. He tells you that he is afraid he might have cancer.

Your physical examination reveals a normal adult pubic hair pattern and no excoriation or infestation in the pubic hair or at the base of the penis. The penis is circumcised and free of rashes, lesions, and discoloration. No tenderness or nodules are noted on palpation. The urinary meatus is located in the mid-glans, and no discharge is revealed on palpation. Inspection of the scrotum reveals an enlarged right scrotum and redness on the scrotal sac, but no lesions. Palpation of the left testicle, epididymis, and spermatic cord reveal no tenderness, nodules, or swelling. Palpation of the right testicle reveals a 2-centimeter, nonmobile, nontender nodule on the anterior portion of the testicle. The left epididymis and spermatic cord are free of tenderness, nodules, and swelling. No red glow is seen on transillumination of the scrotal contents on either side. No bulges are noted in the inguinal or femoral canal.

■ Self-Reflection and Evaluation of Learner Objectives

After you have read Chapter 19 and completed the above review items, please identify to what degree you have met each of the following chapter learning objectives. For those objectives that you have met partially or not at all, you will want to review chapter content for that learning objective(s).

Objective	Very much	Somewhat	Not at all
1. Describe the structure and functions of the male genitalia.			
2. Discuss risk factors for HIV/AIDS and ways to reduce these risk factors.			
3. Discuss the incidence of AIDS across cultures.			
4. Obtain an accurate nursing history of the male client's genitalia.			
5. Explain how to prepare the client for a genitalia examination.			
6. Describe the equipment necessary to perform an examination of the male genitalia.			

(continues)

(Continued)

Objective	Very much	Somewhat	Not at all
7. Inspect the base of the penis and pubic hair for hair growth pattern and the presence of excoriation, erythema, or infestation.			
8. Inspect the skin of the shaft for rashes, lesions, or lumps.			
9. Palpate the shaft for hardened areas or tenderness.			
10. Inspect the foreskin (if present) for color, location, and integrity.			
11. Inspect the glans for size, shape, and presence of lesions or redness.			
12. Palpate for urethral discharge.			
13. Inspect the client's scrotum for size, shape, and position (observe for swelling, lumps, and bulges) and the skin for color, integrity, and the presence of lesions or rashes.			
14. Palpate the client's scrotal sac contents (testes and epididymis) for size, shape, consistency, and presence of tenderness or nodules. Palpate each spermatic cord and vas deferens for nodules, swelling, or tenderness.			
15. Transilluminate the scrotal contents if an abnormal mass or swelling is noted.			
16. Palpate the client's inguinal area for inguinal and femoral hernias.			
17. Palpate for the presence of a scrotal hernia.			
18. Describe changes often seen with aging of the male genitalia.			

For additional information on this book, be sure to visit *http://connection.lww.com.*

CHAPTER 20

Female Genitalia Assessment

CHAPTER OVERVIEW

Like the male genitalia, the female genitalia consist of internal and external structures; and like the male genital assessment, the female genital assessment requires the nurse's tact and sensitivity. The key goals of the assessment are screening and detection of serious or life-threatening problems, such as cervical cancer, and patient education and health promotion. Use the following exercises and quizzes to help you review basic techniques and skills.

■ Multiple Choice Questions

Choose the one best answer for each of the following multiple-choice questions.

_____ 1. The skin folds of the labia majora are composed of adipose tissue, sebaceous glands, and

    A. Skene's ducts.

    B. vestibular glands.

    C. sweat glands.

    D. Bartholin's glands.

_____ 2. The visible portion of the clitoris is termed the

    A. corpus.

    B. crura.

    C. vestibule.

    D. glans.

_____ 3. The skin folds of the labia majora and the labia minora form a boat-shaped area termed the

    A. vestibule.

    B. corpus.

    C. Skene's glands.

    D. urethral meatus.

_____ 4. The outermost layer of the vaginal wall is composed of

    A. pink squamous epithelium and connective tissue.

    B. the vascular supply, nerves, and lymphatic channels.

    C. smooth muscle and connective tissue.

    D. connective tissue and the vascular network.

_____ 5. The outer layer of the vaginal wall is under the direct influence of
    A. androgen.
    B. progesterone.
    C. aldosterone.
    D. estrogen.

LABELING ACTIVITY

Label the following structures of the external female genitalia.

External genitalia

Label the structure indicated by the line; then match your answer with the label on the matching figure in chapter 20 of your textbook.

Label the following structures of the internal female genitalia.

Internal genitalia.

Label the structure indicated by the line; then match your answer with the label on the matching figure in chapter 20 of your textbook.

WORKING WITH PEERS IN LEARNING LAB

After reading Chapter 20, participate in the following learning activities.

1. Review the information in the Risk Factors box in Chapter 20. Determine your own risk for cervical cancer and ways to reduce these risk factors. Next, identify and discuss ethnic groups that are at high risk for cervical cancer.

2. Obtain brochures and literature on cervical cancer and Pap smear testing from the county health department, your campus student health center, or the American Cancer Society. Discuss with your lab partner how to best give a presentation on this topic to teenagers and then to a college-aged group.

3. Using a model of the female genitalia, review the anatomy and function of each anatomic structure. Discuss the assessment findings with your lab partner as they compare with those of an elderly woman.

INTERVIEWING AND RECORDING ASSESSMENT FINDINGS

Because of the sensitive nature of completing a female genitalia assessment, you will want to conduct a nursing history either by using a case study provided by your instructor or by having your lab partner assume the role of a fictitious client to answer the questions. Use the following Nursing History Checklist for your interview.

NURSING HISTORY CHECKLIST

Questions	Normal findings	Abnormal findings	Data missing
Current Symptoms			
1. Menstrual cycles (date of last period, regular cycles, length, describe typical amount of blood flow, symptoms experienced before or during period)?			
2. Age at time of first menstrual period?			
3. Menopause: Stopped menstruating (if yes, at what age?) or having irregular periods? What symptoms experienced?			
4. Vaginal discharge (unusual in color, amount, or odor)?			
5. Pain or itching in genitalia or groin?			
6. Lumps, swelling, or masses in genital area?			
7. Urinating difficulty, change in urine color, or developed an odor? Difficulty controlling urine?			
8. Problems with sexual performance?			
9. Recent change in sexual activity pattern or libido?			
10. Fertility problems now or in the past?			

(continues)

NURSING HISTORY CHECKLIST *(Continued)*

Questions	Normal findings	Abnormal findings	Data missing

Past History

1. Previous gynecologic problems and results of any treatment?

2. Date of last pelvic exam by a physician? Date of last Pap smear? Results?

3. Ever diagnosed with a sexually transmitted disease (STD)? How treated?

4. Past pregnancies? Number of pregnancies? Number of children? Possibility of being pregnant now?

Family History

1. Family history of reproductive or genital cancer? Type? How is the family member related to you?

Lifestyle and Health Practices

1. Do you smoke, or have you smoked in the past? Amount and length of time?

2. Number of sexual partners?

3. Use of contraceptives? Type? Frequency?

4. Problems with your genitalia that affect your functioning?

5. What is your sexual preference?

6. Comfort level communicating with your partner your sexual likes and dislikes?

7. Fears related to sex? Do you have stress related to sex?

8. Fertility concerns? If so, has this affected your relationship with partner or family?

9. Feelings about going through menopause?

10. Do you perform monthly genital self-exams?

11. Tested for HIV? Results? Why tested?

12. Taking estrogen replacement? Length of treatment? Dosage?

13. Knowledge of toxic shock syndrome?

14. Knowledge of sexually transmitted diseases and their prevention?

PERFORMING PHYSICAL ASSESSMENT

Obtain a model of the female reproductive system Use the following Physical Assessment Checklist as your guide to performing a genital assessment.

PHYSICAL ASSESSMENT CHECKLIST

Assessment Skill	Findings (Normal or Abnormal) and Notes		Performance (Satisfactory, Needs Improvement, Unsatisfactory)		
	N	A	S	N	U
1. Gather equipment: stool, light, speculum, emesis basin filled with warm tap water, Surgilube, cotton-tipped applicators, *Chlamydia* culture tube, culturette, test tube with water, sterile gloves, Ayre spatula (wood stick), and feminine napkins.	☐	☐	☐	☐	☐
2. Explain procedure to client.	☐	☐	☐	☐	☐
3. Ask client to gown.	☐	☐	☐	☐	☐
External Genitalia					
1. Inspect the mons pubis. Note pubic hair distribution, signs of infestation.	☐	☐	☐	☐	☐
2. Inspect the labia majora and perineum. Note lesions, swelling, excoriation.	☐	☐	☐	☐	☐
3. Inspect the labia minora, clitoris, urethral meatus, and vaginal opening. Note lesions, excoriation, swelling, discharge.	☐	☐	☐	☐	☐
4. Palpate the Bartholin's glands (if history of swelling or current swelling noted). Note swelling, tenderness, discharge.	☐	☐	☐	☐	☐
5. Palpate the urethra (if client complains of urethral symptoms or urethritis, or inflammation of Skene's glands is suspected) by inserting gloved index finger into the superior portion of the vagina and milking the urethra from the inside, pushing up and out. Observe for drainage.	☐	☐	☐	☐	☐
Internal Genitalia					
1. Inspect the size of the vaginal opening and the angle of the vagina by moistening gloved index finger with warm water and gently inserting the finger into the vagina.	☐	☐	☐	☐	☐
2. Assess the vaginal musculature by keeping index finger inserted in the vaginal opening and asking client to squeeze around your finger. Using middle and index fingers to separate the labia minora, ask client to bear down. Observe for bulging or discharge of urine.	☐	☐	☐	☐	☐
3. Perform the speculum examination:					
a. Inspect the cervix for color, size, position, surface, os, discharge, or lesions.	☐	☐	☐	☐	☐
b. Obtain specimens for the Pap smear and, if indicated, cultures to test for STDs.	☐	☐	☐	☐	☐
c. Inspect the vagina, unlocking the speculum and inspecting the vagina as the partially open speculum is slowly rotated and removed. Note color, surface, consistency, and discharge.	☐	☐	☐	☐	☐

(continues)

PHYSICAL ASSESSMENT CHECKLIST *(Continued)*

Assessment Skill	Findings (Normal or Abnormal) and Notes		Performance (Satisfactory, Needs Improvement, Unsatisfactory)		
	N	A	S	N	U
4. Perform the bimanual examination by placing nondominant hand on lower abdomen and inserting gloved, lubricated, index and middle fingers into the vaginal opening, applying pressure to the posterior wall, and waiting for the opening to relax. Palpate the ovaries by sliding your intravaginal fingers to the right lateral fornix and attempting to palpate the left and then right ovaries. Note size, shape, consistency, mobility, and tenderness. Observe for secretions as fingers are withdrawn.	☐	☐	☐	☐	☐
5. Perform the rectovaginal examination by changing gloves on dominant hand and lubricating index and middle fingers. Ask client to bear down. Insert index finger into the vagina and middle finger into the rectum. While pushing down on the abdominal wall with the other hand, palpate the internal reproductive structures through the anterior rectal wall, with attention to the area behind the cervix, the rectovaginal septum, the cul-de-sac, and the posterior uterine wall.	☐	☐	☐	☐	☐
Analysis of Data					
1. Formulate nursing diagnoses (wellness, risk, actual).	☐	☐	☐	☐	☐
2. Formulate collaborative problems.	☐	☐	☐	☐	☐
3. Make necessary referrals.	☐	☐	☐	☐	☐

CRITICAL THINKING AND CASE STUDIES

1. Develop a seminar on prevention of sexually transmitted disease (STD) for a group of college freshmen.

2. What variations of the cervix are considered normal?

3. Compare and contrast how you would focus the nursing history of the female genitalia for an 18-year-old versus that for an 80-year-old.

4. Read the following case study. Develop possible nursing diagnoses that are appropriate for this client:

Ann Smith, 37, has made an appointment with the OB/GYN nurse practitioner. You are asked to compile the nursing history. When you ask Mrs. Smith why she is here today, she looks somewhat embarrassed and answers quietly, "I am having trouble with sexual intercourse." She goes on to explain that she has had decreased interest in sex, and her vagina seems drier than usual. When asked whether she has been able to discuss this problem with her husband, she says, "No . . . it is embarrassing . . . we have always enjoyed sex, and I feel I am not meeting his needs any more. I can tell he is getting very frustrated. He asks me why we never have sex any more, and I just give excuses of having headaches, being tired, or being too busy."

You ask her what is going on in her life right now, and Ann tells you that she is under a lot of stress at her marketing job and that lately she has had to help her two kids, aged 10 and 8, with a lot of school projects. She is also worried about her mother, who is undergoing tests to determine whether she has cancer.

5. On the basis of the following assessment information, work through the steps of analyzing the data. Identify abnormal data and strengths in **subjective and objective findings**, assemble **cue clusters**, draw **inferences**, make possible **nursing diagnoses**, identify **defining characteristics, confirm or rule out** the nursing diagnosis, and **document** your conclusions.

   Use the blank diagnostic analysis charts provided at the end of this book to guide your thinking. You may want to write on the chart or use separate paper. Propose nursing diagnoses that are specific to the client in the case study. Identify collaborative problems, if any, for this client. Finally, identify data, if any, that point toward a medical problem requiring a referral.

   Tina Kehler is a 26-year-old white woman. She is a single mother of two and is employed as a paralegal in a law firm. She comes to the clinic appearing anxious. She states she is experiencing a brown vaginal discharge that started 2 days ago. When interviewed, she states that her last pelvic examination was 6 months ago. She denies any history of cancer or abnormal Pap smear results. Her last menstrual period was normal and ended 1 week ago today. She has never been tested for HIV. She admits to unprotected sex 3 weeks ago with her boyfriend. A Norplant birth control device was placed in her left arm 1 year ago. Tina denies smoking, states that she doesn't follow any special diet, and doesn't exercise on a regular basis. She explains that she is not comfortable discussing this problem with her new boyfriend—"I am afraid he might leave me."

   Your physical assessment reveals normal hair distribution and no lesions, masses, or swelling. The labia majora and labia minora are pink, moist, and free of lesions, excoriation, and swelling. A small amount of malodorous brown discharge is noted at the vaginal orifice. There is no bulging at vaginal orifice. The perineum is intact, with a healed episiotomy scar. No discharge is observed on urethral palpation. Internal examination reveals cervix to be slightly anterior and pink, with a slit-like os, and free of lesions. A brown discharge is noted on the cervix. The vaginal walls are pink and moist, with streaks of brown discharge. Bimanual examination reveals a mobile, firm, but tender cervix. The fundus is palpated at the level of the symphysis pubis. The ovaries are palpated bilaterally without lesions and are approximately 3 centimeters. The right ovary is very tender on palpation. A routine Pap smear is performed, and culture specimens are taken. A smooth, firm, mobile, nontender posterior uterine wall and a smooth, firm, thin, movable rectovaginal septum are palpated during rectovaginal palpation.

■ Chapter Post-test

MULTIPLE CHOICE QUESTIONS

Choose the one best answer for each of the following multiple-choice questions.

_____ 1. A female client tells the nurse that she may be experiencing premenstrual syndrome. An appropriate question for the nurse to ask the client is

    A. "How often are your menstrual periods?"

    B. "Do you experience mood swings or bloating?"

    C. "Are you experiencing regular menstrual cycles?"

    D. "How old were you when you began to menstruate?"

_____ 2. A 53-year-old client tells the nurse that she thinks she is starting the menopausal phase of her life. The nurse should instruct the client that she may experience

    A. hot flashes.

    B. increased appetite.

    C. vaginal discharge.

    D. urinary frequency.

_____ 3. During assessment of the vaginal area of an adult client, the client tells the nurse that she has had pain in her vaginal area. The nurse should further assess the client for

    A. trauma.

    B. cancer.

    C. pregnancy.

    D. infection.

_____ 4. A female client tells the nurse that she has pain while urinating. Besides obtaining a urinalysis, the nurse should assess the client for

    A. kidney trauma.

    B. sexually transmitted disease.

    C. tumors.

    D. infestation.

_____ 5. An older adult client visits the clinic complaining of urinary incontinence. The nurse should explain to the client that this is often due to

    A. decreased urethral elasticity.

    B. atrophy of the vaginal mucosa.

    C. change in the vaginal pH.

    D. decreased estrogen production.

_____ 6. A female client has scheduled a physical examination, including a Pap smear. The nurse should instruct the client to

    A. refrain from douching 48 hours before the examination.

    B. bring in a urine sample for testing.

C. drink a large volume of fluid before the examination.

D. refrain from using talcum powder after her shower.

_____ 7. The nurse is preparing to perform a speculum examination on an adult woman. To lubricate the speculum before insertion, the nurse should use

A. sterile water.

B. K-Y jelly.

C. warm tap water.

D. petroleum jelly.

_____ 8. The nurse is performing a speculum examination on an adult woman. The nurse is having difficulty inserting the speculum because the client is unable to relax. The nurse should ask the client to

A. bear down.

B. hold her breath.

C. use imagery to relax.

D. take a deep breath.

_____ 9. The nurse is assessing the genitalia of a female client and detects a bulging anterior wall in the vagina. The nurse should plan to refer the client to a physician for

A. stress incontinence.

B. rectocele.

C. tumor of the vagina.

D. cystocele.

_____ 10. An older adult client visits the clinic for a gynecologic examination. The client tells the nurse that she has been told that she has uterine prolapse. The nurse should further assess the client for

A. stress incontinence.

B. cystocele.

C. a retroverted uterus.

D. diastasis recti.

_____ 11. While assessing the cervix of an adult client, the nurse observes a yellowish discharge from the cervix. The nurse should further assess the client for a/an

A. infection.

B. abnormal lesion.

C. positive pregnancy test result.

D. polyp.

_____ 12. While performing a gynecologic examination, the nurse observes small, painful, ulcer-like lesions with red bases on the client's labia. The nurse should refer the client to a physician for possible

A. herpes simplex virus infection.

B. syphilis.

C. lice.

D. herpes zoster virus infection.

_____ 13. While assessing the genitalia of a female client, the nurse observes moist, fleshy lesions on the client's labia. The nurse should refer the client to a physician for possible

   A. gonorrhea.

   B. herpes simplex virus infection.

   C. nabothian cysts.

   D. genital warts.

_____ 14. During a gynecologic examination, the nurse observes that the client has a yellow-green frothy vaginal discharge. The nurse should plan to test the client for possible

   A. _Trichomonas vaginalis_ infection.

   B. bacterial vaginosis.

   C. atrophic vaginitis.

   D. _Chlamydia trachomatis_ infection.

_____ 15. A client visits the clinic because she has missed one period and suspects she is pregnant. While assessing the client, the nurse detects a solid, mobile, tender unilateral adnexal mass. The client's cervix is soft. The nurse suspects that the client may be experiencing

   A. normal pregnancy.

   B. endometriosis.

   C. pelvic inflammatory disease.

   D. ectopic pregnancy.

MATCHING

Match the terms in the left column with the correct description in the right column.

Term	Description
_____ 1. Skene's glands	A. Painful menstruation
_____ 2. Bartholin's glands	B. Cessation of menstruation
_____ 3. Os	C. "Crabs"
_____ 4. Libido	D. Heavy menstruation
_____ 5. Pediculosis pubis	E. Secrete mucus to aid in lubrication during intercourse
_____ 6. Chadwick's sign	F. Desire for sexual activity
_____ 7. Mons pubis	G. Secrete mucus to lubricate and maintain moist vaginal environment
_____ 8. Menopause	H. Cervix appears blue rather than pink
_____ 9. Amenorrhea	I. Painful urination
_____ 10. Menorrhagia	J. Absence of menstruation
_____ 11. Dysmenorrhea	K. Opening in center of cervix
_____ 12. Dysuria	L. Round, firm pad of adipose tissue that covers the symphysis pubis

■ Self-Reflection and Evaluation of Learner Objectives

After you have read Chapter 20 and completed the above review items, please identify to what degree you have met each of the following chapter learning objectives. For any objective that you have met partially or not at all, you will want to review chapter content for that learning objective.

Objective	Very much	Somewhat	Not at all
1. Describe the structure and functions of the female genitalia.			
2. Discuss risk factors for cervical cancer and ways to reduce these risk factors.			
3. Discuss the incidence of cervical cancer across cultures.			
4. Obtain an accurate nursing history of the female client's genitalia.			
5. Explain how to prepare the client for a genitalia examination.			
6. Describe the equipment necessary to perform an examination of the female genitalia.			
7. Assess the external genitalia by inspecting the mons pubis for pubic hair distribution and perineum for lesions, swelling, and excoriation.			
8. Inspect the labia minora, clitoris, urethral meatus, and vaginal opening for lesions, excoriation, swelling, and discharge.			
9. Palpate the Bartholin's glands (if labia swelling noted or a history of swelling) noting swelling, tenderness, and discharge.			
10. Palpate the urethra if the client has urethral complaints or symptoms.			
11. Assess the internal female genitalia by inspecting the size of the vaginal opening, the angle of the vagina, and the vaginal musculature.			
12. Assess the internal female genitalia, using the speculum to inspect the vagina for color, size, position, surface, os, consistency, discharge, and lesions.			
13. Perform the bimanual examination of the vaginal wall, assessing for texture and tenderness and palpating the cervix for contour, consistency, mobility, and tenderness.			
14. Palpate the client's uterus for position, shape, and consistency.			
15. Palpate the client's ovaries for size, shape, consistency, mobility, and tenderness.			
16. Perform the rectovaginal examination to assess the rectovaginal septum and posterior uterine wall.			

For additional information on this book, be sure to visit *http://connection.lww.com*.

CHAPTER 21

Anus, Rectum, and Prostate Assessment

CHAPTER OVERVIEW

The anus and rectum complete the gastrointestinal tract. In men, the prostate gland is integrally entwined with these structures. In both men and women, the colon is also examined during assessment of the rectum and the anus. The assessment is particularly important for detecting signs and symptoms of colon cancer; prostatic conditions, which affect most older men; and other intestinal disorders.

■ Chapter Pretest

MULTIPLE CHOICE

Choose the one best answer for each of the following multiple-choice questions.

_____ 1. The external sphincter of the anus is
   A. composed of smooth muscle.
   B. composed of skeletal muscle.
   C. composed of striated muscle.
   D. under involuntary control.

_____ 2. The external sphincter and internal sphincter of the rectum are divided by the
   A. anorectal junction.
   B. rectovesical pouch.
   C. median sulcus.
   D. intersphincteric groove.

_____ 3. The rectum is lined with folds of mucosa, and each fold contains a network of arteries, veins, and visceral nerves. When these veins undergo chronic pressure, the result may be
   A. polyps.
   B. tumors.
   C. fissures.
   D. hemorrhoids.

_____ 4. The prostate gland consists of two lobes separated by the
   A. median sulcus.
   B. rectovesical pouch.

    C. anorectal junction.

    D. valves of Houston.

_____ 5. The prostate functions to

    A. store sperm until ejaculation occurs.

    B. secrete a milky substance that neutralizes female acidic secretions.

    C. produce the ejaculate that nourishes and protects sperm.

    D. produce mucus-like fluid to assist in lubrication.

_____ 6. The Cowper's glands

    A. are located inside the rectum.

    B. produce a substance to aid in sperm motility.

    C. empty into the urethra.

    D. can be palpated through the rectum.

LABELING ACTIVITY

Label the following structures of the anus and rectum.

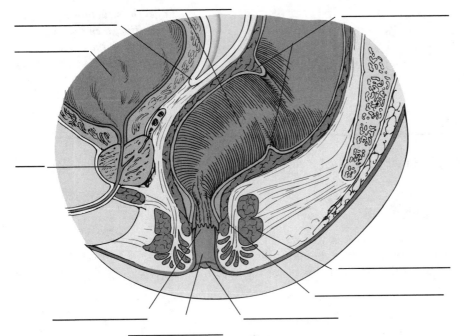

Anus and rectum.

Label the structure indicated by the line; then match your answer with the label on the matching figure in chapter 21 of your textbook.

Label the following parts of the prostate gland.

Prostate.

Label the structure indicated by the line; then match your answer with the label on the matching figure in chapter 21 of your textbook.

■ Learner Activities

After reading Chapter 21, participate in the following learning activities.

WORKING WITH PEERS IN LEARNING LAB

1. Review the information in the Risk Factors box in Chapter 21. Determine your own risk for colorectal cancer and ways to reduce these risk factors. Next, identify and discuss the ethnic groups that are at high risk for this type of cancer.

2. Obtain brochures and literature from the county health department, a local health care facility, or the American Cancer Society. Discuss with your lab partner the best way to approach a presentation on this topic to a group of middle-aged men and women.

3. Obtain brochures and literature from the county health department, a local health care facility, or the American Cancer Society about prostate cancer. Discuss with your lab partner how best to present this topic to a group of men. Talk about how you might handle discussing this potentially sensitive topic.

4. Using a model of the anus, rectum, and prostate, review the anatomy and function of each anatomic structure. Discuss the assessment findings with your lab partner as they compare with those of an older person.

INTERVIEWING AND RECORDING ASSESSMENT FINDINGS

Because of the sensitive nature of completing an assessment of the anus, rectum, and prostate, you will want to conduct a nursing history either by using either a case study provided by your instructor or by having your lab partner assume the role of a fictitious client to answer the questions. Use the following Nursing History Checklist as a guide to interviewing and recording your findings.

NURSING HISTORY CHECKLIST

Questions	Normal findings	Abnormal findings	Additional data needed
Current Symptoms			
1. Problems with bowels (bowel pattern changes, constipation, diarrhea, bowel control, stool color, blood or mucus in stool, pain or itching in rectal area, hemorrhoids)?			
2. Anal and perianal problems (lumps, ulcers, lesions, rashes, redness)?			
3. Sacrococcygeal area (pilonidal) swelling, redness, dimpling, or hair?			
4. Frequent nighttime urination?			
Past History			
1. Previous anal or rectal trauma or surgery, congenital deformities?			
2. History of blood in stool?			
3. History of prostate enlargement, treatment or urgery on the prostate?			
4. Pattern of health screenings (occult blood, prostate-specific antigen, procto-sigmoidoscopy, colonoscopy)?			
Lifestyle and Health Practices			
1. Use of laxatives, stool softeners, enemas, or other bowel medications?			
2. Practice anal sex?			
3. Daily water/fluid intake?			
4. Usual diet (high fiber and roughage, saturated fat content)?			
5. Usual exercise pattern?			
6. Any effect on daily life from anal, rectal, or bowel problems, or from prostate problems?			

PERFORMING PHYSICAL ASSESSMENT

Use the following Physical Assessment Checklist as your guide to performing an assessment of the anus, rectum, and prostate gland.

PHYSICAL ASSESSMENT CHECKLIST

Assessment Skill	Findings (Normal or Abnormal) and Notes		Performance (Satisfactory, Needs Improvement, Unsatisfactory)		
	N	A	S	N	U
1. Gather equipment (gloves, lubricating gel).	☐	☐	☐	☐	☐
2. Explain procedure to client.	☐	☐	☐	☐	☐
3. Ask client to gown.	☐	☐	☐	☐	☐
Anus and Perianal Area					
1. Inspect for lumps, ulcers, lesions, rashes, redness (note size, shape, location, distribution, and configuration).	☐	☐	☐	☐	☐
2. Inspect sacrococcygeal area for swelling, redness, dimpling, or presence of hair in pilonidal area.	☐	☐	☐	☐	☐
3. Inspect for rectal prolapse with Valsalva maneuver.	☐	☐	☐	☐	☐
4. Palpate for anal sphincter tone, tenderness, nodules, or hardness.	☐	☐	☐	☐	☐
Rectum and Prostate					
1. Palpate rectal mucosa for tenderness, irregularities, nodules, and hardness.	☐	☐	☐	☐	☐
2. Palpate peritoneal cavity for tenderness or nodules, or "rectal shelf."	☐	☐	☐	☐	☐
3. For males, palpate the prostate gland for tenderness, size, shape, texture, or irregularities.	☐	☐	☐	☐	☐
4. Inspect the feces for blood, and perform occult blood test.	☐	☐	☐	☐	☐
Analysis of Data					
1. Formulate nursing diagnoses (wellness, risk, actual).	☐	☐	☐	☐	☐
2. Formulate collaborative problems.	☐	☐	☐	☐	☐
3. Make necessary referrals.	☐	☐	☐	☐	☐

CRITICAL THINKING AND CASE STUDIES

1. Describe your communication techniques, nursing history questions, and physical examination of the anus, rectum, and prostate for a 26-year-old man who engages in anal sex. Include what and how you would teach about the risk factors for various diseases or conditions.

2. Read the following case study. Develop possible appropriate nursing diagnoses and collaborative problems for Mrs. Cohen.

   Mrs. Cohen is 85 years old. She has a long history of chronic constipation, internal and external hemorrhoids, and heavy use of laxatives. She describes another bout of constipation with no bowel movement for 5 days, but with a feeling of fullness in her rectum. She says that she eats many vegetables when she feels better, but gets too weak to cook or exercise, or even to get dressed, when she has these bouts of constipation. On examination, you note internal and external hemorrhoids, a moderate amount of hard, formed stool in the rectum, and an area of hardness and irregularity about 2 cm in size in the distal portion of the rectum. The results of her stool test are positive for occult blood.

3. On the basis of the following assessment information, work through the steps of analyzing the data. Identify abnormal data and strengths in **subjective and objective findings**, assemble **cue clusters**, draw **inferences**, make possible **nursing diagnoses**, identify **defining characteristics**, **confirm or rule out** the nursing diagnosis, and **document** your conclusions.

   Use the blank diagnostic analysis charts provided at the end of this book to guide your thinking. You may want to write on the chart or use separate paper. Propose nursing diagnoses that are specific to the client in the case study. Identify collaborative problems, if any, for this client. Finally, identify data, if any, that point toward a medical problem requiring a referral.

   Jim Czerniski, a 35-year-old white man, arrives at his primary care provider's office for his annual physical examination. At the start of the interview, he says to you, "My wife is a nurse and she makes me have a physical examination every year—especially with my family history." On questioning, you discover that his father died 4 years ago from colon cancer and that his brother has undergone three biopsies of rectal polyps. Mr. Czerniski states that he has undergone two rectal polyp biopsies, one last year and one 3 years ago. He denies recent changes in his bowel habits and has not noticed any blood in his stool. Jim looks a bit embarrassed when you ask how much water he drinks and how much fiber and roughage he eats. "I know I am supposed to eat a high-fiber diet and drink lots of water—my wife and I get in fights about it. I try real hard, but I am a Big Mac kinda guy, ya know? I eat what my wife fixes me for dinner, but I eat fast food for breakfast and lunch."

   Your physical examination reveals a moist, hairless anal opening with a tightly closed external sphincter. The perianal area is free of redness, lumps, ulcers, lesions, and rashes. No bulging or lesions appear when the client performs the Valsalva maneuver. The sacrococcygeal area is smooth and free of redness and hair. During palpation, the client can close the external sphincter around your gloved finger. The anus feels smooth and is free of nodules and hardness. The client reports that he feels no tenderness. As you palpate farther up in the rectum, you can just detect a small, soft nodule on the rectal wall. The client says he feels no tenderness. Palpation of the peritoneal cavity area reveals a smooth, nontender surface. The prostate gland is palpated as two smooth lobes, 2.5-centimeters long. They feel rubbery and are nontender. The median sulcus is palpated between the two lobes. When you withdraw your hand, you notice a small amount of semisolid brown stool on your glove. You send the stool to be tested for occult blood.

▪ Chapter Post-test

MULTIPLE CHOICE QUESTIONS

Choose the one best answer for each of the following multiple-choice questions.

_____ 1. A client visits the clinic and tells the nurse that she has had "runny diarrhea" for 2 days. The nurse should assess the client for

   A. gastrointestinal infection.

   B. fecal impaction.

   C. constipation.

   D. hemorrhoids.

_____ 2. A client visits the clinic and tells the nurse that his stools have been black for the past 3 days. The nurse should assess the client for

   A. gallbladder disease.

   B. colitis.

   C. polyps.

   D. gastrointestinal bleeding.

_____ 3. A client visits the clinic and tells the nurse that his stools have been pale for the past 2 days and his skin has been itching. The nurse should refer the client to a physician for possible

   A. biliary disease.

   B. cancer.

   C. gastrointestinal infection.

   D. hemorrhoids.

_____ 4. The nurse has instructed a 55-year-old male client about the need for a stool test for occult blood. The nurse determines that the client understands the instructions when he says the test should be performed every

   A. year.

   B. 2 years.

   C. 3 years.

   D. 4 years.

_____ 5. The nurse is planning a presentation on the topic of colorectal cancer to a group of older adults. Which of the following should the nurse plan to include in the presentation?

   A. Colorectal cancer rates have steadily fallen over the past 30 years.

   B. 80% of those diagnosed with colorectal cancer are younger than 50 years of age.

   C. Diets high in fat and low in fiber are associated with colorectal cancer.

   D. Colorectal cancer rates are decreasing outside the United States.

_____ 6. A 60-year-old male client asks the nurse about risk factors for prostate cancer. The nurse should explain to the client that one possible risk factor is

   A. a high-carbohydrate diet.

   B. exposure to sulfur.

    C. genetic inheritance.

    D. advanced age.

_____ 7. Cultural factors play an important role in the development of prostate cancer in men. Which culture has the highest prostate cancer rate?

    A. African-American

    B. white American

    C. Italian

    D. Japanese

_____ 8. The nurse is planning to assess the anus and rectum of an adult male client. The nurse should position the client in a

    A. right lateral position.

    B. left lateral position.

    C. prone position.

    D. knee-chest position.

_____ 9. The nurse is planning to inspect the anal area of an adult male client. To assess for any bulges or lesions, the nurse should ask the client to

    A. hold his breath.

    B. breathe deeply through his mouth.

    C. breathe normally.

    D. bear down.

_____ 10. While assessing the anal area of an adult client, the nurse detects redness and excoriation. The nurse determines that this sign is most likely due to

    A. internal hemorrhoids.

    B. an anorectal fistula.

    C. a fungal infection.

    D. previous surgery.

_____ 11. While assessing the anal area of an adult client, the nurse observes a reddened, swollen area covered by a small tuft of hair located midline on the lower sacrum. The nurse should refer the client to a physician for possible

    A. perianal abscess.

    B. neurologic disorder.

    C. pilonidal cyst.

    D. anorectal fistula.

_____ 12. While assessing the anus of an adult client, the nurse detects the presence of small nodules. The nurse should refer the client to a physician for possible

    A. polyps.

    B. anorectal fistula.

    C. hemorrhoids.

    D. rectocele.

_____ 13. While assessing the anus of an adult client, the nurse detects a peritoneal protrusion. The nurse should refer the client to a physician for possible

    A. anorectal fistula.

    B. polyps.

    C. prostate enlargement.

    D. peritoneal metastasis.

_____ 14. While examining the prostate gland of an older adult, the nurse detects hard, fixed nodules. The nurse should refer the client to a physician for possible

    A. prostate cancer.

    B. benign prostatic hypertrophy.

    C. acute prostatitis.

    D. prostatocystitis.

MATCHING

Match the terms in the left column with the correct descriptions in the right column.

Term	Description
_____ 1. Constipation	A. Three semilunar transverse folds within the rectal interior
_____ 2. Diarrhea	B. Examination of the rectum and sigmoid colon with the sigmoidoscope
_____ 3. Hemorrhoids	C. Client holds the breath and bears down
_____ 4. Pilonidal cyst	D. Frequent, loose stools
_____ 5. Prostate-specific antigen (PSA) test	E. Medicines that loosen the bowel contents and encourage evacuation
_____ 6. Proctosigmoidoscopy	F. Infrequent, hard stool
_____ 7. Colonoscopy	G. Excessive fat in the stool
_____ 8. Laxatives	H. Blood test to detect prostate cancer
_____ 9. Enema	I. Endoscopic examination of the colon, either transabdominally during laparotomy, or transanally by colonoscopy
_____ 10. Valsalva maneuver	J. A hair-containing cyst located in the midline over the coccyx or lower sacrum
_____ 11. Valves of Houston	K. A solution introduced into the rectum to promote evacuation of feces
_____ 12. Steatorrhea	L. Painless, flabby papules due to varicose veins; two types, external or internal

■ Self-Reflection and Evaluation of Learner Objectives

After you have read Chapter 21 and completed the above quizzes and activities, please identify to what degree you have met each of the following chapter learning objectives. For those objectives that you have met partially or not at all, you will want to review chapter content for that learning objective.

Objective	Very much	Somewhat	Not at all
1. Describe the structures and function of the anus and rectum.			
2. Discuss the risk factors for colorectal cancer and ways to reduce these risk factors.			
3. Discuss the incidence of colorectal cancer across the cultures.			
4. Describe the structures and functions of the prostate.			
5. Discuss risk factors for prostate cancer and ways to reduce these risk factors.			
6. Discuss the incidence of prostate cancer across the cultures.			
7. Obtain an accurate history of the client's anus, rectum, and prostate health.			
8. Explain how to prepare the client for an examination of the anus, rectum, and prostate.			
9. Describe special care to be used with assessment of the anus, rectum, and prostate.			
10. Describe the equipment necessary to perform an assessment of the anus, rectum, and prostate.			
11. Describe the two physical examination techniques (inspection and palpation) used to assess the anus, rectum, and prostate.			
12. Inspect the perianal area for lumps, ulcers, lesions, rashes, or redness (p. 483) and the sacrococcygeal area for swelling, redness, dimpling, or hair.			
13. Palpate the anus for sphincter tone, tenderness or pain, nodules, and hardness.			
14. Palpate the rectum for tenderness, irregularities, nodules, or hardness.			
15. Palpate the peritoneal cavity and prostate (males) for tenderness or nodules.			
16. Inspect stool for color and consistency; also test for occult blood.			
17. Discuss various nursing diagnoses and collaborative problems commonly seen with assessment of the anus, rectum, and prostate.			

For additional information on this book, be sure to visit *http://connection.lww.com*.

CHAPTER 22

Musculoskeletal Assessment

CHAPTER OVERVIEW

Muscles, bones, joints, ligaments, and tendons are the body's infrastructure—
the elements that allow humans an upright posture and extensive mobility.
Changes that occur in other body systems may have a profound effect on the
musculoskeletal system, and changes that occur in the musculoskeletal system
itself affect the activities of daily living and quality of life across the life span,
making careful and accurate assessment extremely important.

■ Chapter Pretest

MULTIPLE CHOICE

Choose the one best answer for each of the following multiple-choice questions.

_____ 1. One of the functions of a bone is to
   A. store fat.
   B. produce secretions.
   C. produce blood cells.
   D. store protein.

_____ 2. Bones contain yellow marrow that is composed mainly of
   A. fat.
   B. protein.
   C. cartilage.
   D. carbohydrates.

_____ 3. The part of a bone that covers the bone and contains osteoblasts and
   blood vessels is termed the
   A. cartilage.
   B. synovial membrane.
   C. connective tissue.
   D. periosteum.

_____ 4. Skeletal muscles are attached to bones by
   A. tendons.
   B. cartilage.
   C. fibrous connective tissue.
   D. ligaments.

_____ 5. Joints may be classified as cartilaginous, synovial, or
   A. articulate.
   B. flexible.
   C. immobile.
   D. fibrous.

_____ 6. Bones in synovial joints are joined together by
   A. cartilage.
   B. ligaments.
   C. tendons.
   D. periosteal tissue.

_____ 7. When the nurse moves the client's arm away from the midline of the body, the nurse is performing
   A. adduction.
   B. external rotation.
   C. retraction.
   D. abduction.

_____ 8. When the nurse moves a client's leg upward, the nurse is performing
   A. supination.
   B. external rotation.
   C. eversion.
   D. internal rotation.

_____ 9. The subacromial bursae are contained in the
   A. temporomandibular joint.
   B. shoulder joint.
   C. elbow joint.
   D. wrist joint.

_____ 10. Articulation between the head of the femur and the acetabulum is in the
   A. knee joint.
   B. tibial joint.
   C. ankle joint.
   D. hip joint.

LABELING ACTIVITY

Label the major bones and joints of the shoulder and elbow.

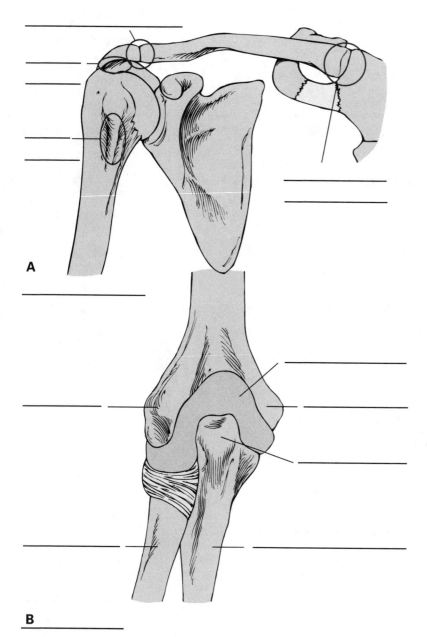

(A) Sternoclavicular joint.
(B) Elbow.

Label the structure indicated by the line; then match your answer with the label on the matching figure in chapter 22 of your textbook.

Label the major bones and joints of the hip and knee.

(A) Hip
(B) Knee.

Label the structure indicated by the line; then match your answer with the label on the matching figure in chapter 22 of your textbook.

■ Learner Activities

After reading Chapter 22, participate in the following learning activities.

WORKING WITH PEERS IN LEARNING LAB

1. Review the information in the Risk Factors box in Chapter 22. Determine your own risk for osteoporosis and ways to reduce these risk factors. Next, identify and discuss the ethnic groups that are at high risk for osteoporosis.

2. Obtain brochures and literature on osteoporosis from the county health department or your local health care facility for information. Discuss with your lab partner how best to give a presentation on this topic to college-aged women and then to a group of middle-aged women.

3. Find an elderly client, friend, or relative who will let you assess his or her musculoskeletal system. With your lab partner, discuss the assessment findings and compare them with the findings from an assessment of a younger person.

INTERVIEWING AND RECORDING ASSESSMENT FINDINGS

Use the following Nursing History Checklist as your guide to interviewing and recording musculoskeletal assessment findings.

NURSING HISTORY CHECKLIST

Questions	Normal findings	Abnormal findings	Additional data needed
Current Symptoms			
1. Recent weight gain			
2. Difficulty chewing			
3. Joint, muscle, or bone throbbing			
Past History			
1. Past problems or injuries to joints, muscles, or bones			
2. Past treatment: surgery, medications, physical therapy, exercise, rest			
3. Tetanus and polio immunizations			
4. Diagnosed with diabetes mellitus, lupus, or sickle-cell anemia			
5. How old at start of menstruation; started menopause; estrogen replacement therapy			
Family History			
1. Family history of rheumatoid arthritis, gout, osteoporosis, psoriasis, infectious tuberculosis			

NURSING HISTORY CHECKLIST

Questions	Normal findings	Abnormal findings	Additional data needed
Lifestyle and Health Practices			
1. Activities to promote musculoskeletal health			
2. Home remedies to relieve musculoskeletal problems			
3. Assistive devices to promote mobility			
4. Smoking			
5. Alcohol or caffeinated beverages			
6. Typical diet-drink milk, take calcium supplements			
7. Occupation			
8. Time in sunlight			
9. Routine exercise			
10. Difficulty with ADLs			
11. Typical posture.			
12. Interference with sexual activities			
13. Ability to interact/socialize			
14. Body Image			
15. Stress			

PERFORMING PHYSICAL ASSESSMENT

Use the following Physical Assessment Checklist as your guide to performing a musculoskeletal assessment.

PHYSICAL ASSESSMENT CHECKLIST

Assessment Skill	Findings (Normal or Abnormal) and Notes		Performance (Satisfactory, Needs Improvement, Unsatisfactory)		
	N	A	S	N	U
1. Gather equipment (tape measure, goniometer).	☐	☐	☐	☐	☐
2. Explain procedure to client.	☐	☐	☐	☐	☐
3. Ask client to gown.	☐	☐	☐	☐	☐
Gait					
1. Observe gait for base, weight-bearing stability, feet position, stride, arm swing, and posture.	☐	☐	☐	☐	☐
Temporomandibular Joint					
1. Inspect, palpate, and test ROM.	☐	☐	☐	☐	☐
Sternoclavicular Joint					
1. Inspect and palpate for midline location, color, swelling, and masses.	☐	☐	☐	☐	☐
Spine					
1. Inspect and palpate cervical, thoracic, and lumbar spine for pain and tenderness.	☐	☐	☐	☐	☐
2. Test ROM of cervical spine.	☐	☐	☐	☐	☐
3. Test ROM of thoracic and lumbar spine.	☐	☐	☐	☐	☐
4. Test for leg and back pain.	☐	☐	☐	☐	☐
5. Measure leg length.	☐	☐	☐	☐	☐
Shoulders					
1. Inspect and palpate shoulders for symmetry, color, swelling, and masses.	☐	☐	☐	☐	☐
2. Test ROM of shoulders.	☐	☐	☐	☐	☐
Elbows					
1. Inspect and palpate elbows for size, shape, deformities, redness, or swelling.	☐	☐	☐	☐	☐
2. Test ROM of elbows.	☐	☐	☐	☐	☐
Wrists					
1. Inspect and palpate wrists for size, shape, symmetry, color, swelling, tenderness, and nodules.	☐	☐	☐	☐	☐
2. Test ROM of wrists.	☐	☐	☐	☐	☐
3. Test for carpal tunnel syndrome.	☐	☐	☐	☐	☐
Hands and Fingers					
1. Inspect and palpate hands and fingers for size, shape, symmetry, swelling, color, tenderness, and nodules.	☐	☐	☐	☐	☐
2. Test ROM of hands and fingers.	☐	☐	☐	☐	☐
Hips					
1. Inspect and palpate hips for shape and symmetry.	☐	☐	☐	☐	☐
2. Test ROM of hips.	☐	☐	☐	☐	☐

PHYSICAL ASSESSMENT CHECKLIST

Assessment Skill	Findings (Normal or Abnormal) and Notes		Performance (Satisfactory, Needs Improvement, Unsatisfactory)		
	N	A	S	N	U
Knees					
1. Inspect and palpate knees for size, shape, symmetry, deformities, pain, and alignment.	☐	☐	☐	☐	☐
2. Test knees for swelling. If small amount of fluid present, do "bulge test." If large amount of fluid present, do "ballottement test."	☐	☐	☐	☐	☐
3. Test ROM of knees.	☐	☐	☐	☐	☐
4. Perform McMurray's test if client complains of "clicking" in knee.	☐	☐	☐	☐	☐
Ankles and Feet					
1. Inspect and palpate ankles and feet for position, alignment, shape, skin, tenderness, temperature, swelling, or nodules.	☐	☐	☐	☐	☐
2. Test ROM of ankles and toes.	☐	☐	☐	☐	☐
Analysis of Data					
1. Formulate nursing diagnoses (wellness, risk, actual).	☐	☐	☐	☐	☐
2. Formulate collaborative problems.	☐	☐	☐	☐	☐
3. Make necessary referrals.	☐	☐	☐	☐	☐

CRITICAL THINKING AND CASE STUDIES

1. Compare and contrast how you would assess for muscle strength, gait, and
   stability in a 25-year-old client versus those in a 75-year-old client.

2. Analyze the following client's risk for osteoporosis.
   A 52-year-old Caucasian woman, married, with two children, is 5 feet 8 inches tall and weighs 130
   pounds. She quit smoking 15 years ago, drinks a lot of milk, went through final stages of menopause 1
   year ago, and is thinking about using hormone (estrogen) replacement therapy.

3. On the basis of the following assessment information, work through the steps
   of analyzing the data. Identify abnormal data and strengths in **subjective and
   objective findings**, assemble **cue clusters**, draw **inferences**, make possible
   nursing diagnoses, identify **defining characteristics, confirm or rule out** the
   nursing diagnosis, and **document** your conclusions.
       Use the blank diagnostic analysis charts provided at the end of this book to
   guide your thinking. You may want to write on the chart or use separate paper.
   Propose nursing diagnoses that are specific to the client in the case study.
   Identify collaborative problems, if any, for this client. Finally, identify data, if
   any, that point toward a medical problem requiring a referral.

   Mrs. Clement is a 71-year-old woman who has had diabetes mellitus for 15
   years. Her diabetes is controlled by diet and insulin. A retired schoolteacher,
   she has lived alone for the past 7 years since her husband died of liver cancer.
   Living in the upper level of a two-story apartment, she socializes with her
   neighbor and regularly attends church. She has a grown son and daughter, who

both live out of state and call frequently but can visit only once a year. Because of her poor eyesight, her neighbor, a retired R.N., helps her draw up her insulin. When visited by the home health care nurse, Mrs. Clement states that she has had lower back and wrist pain for the past month.

During the interview, Mrs. Clement describes a sedentary lifestyle, spending much of her time watching TV, crocheting, or doing crossword puzzles. She uses a magnifying glass for close work. However, she has reduced her handwork because she has been having numbness and tingling in her right thumb and index finger. The pain is relieved by rest, but she often has sharp pain in the right wrist during the night. Mrs. Clement has never smoked, does not drink alcohol, and has five cups of coffee a day. She does little cooking. Her diet primarily consists of TV dinners and canned soups, vegetables, and fruits, with very few dairy products. She reports that constipation has become a more frequent problem over the past month. She has maintained her weight of 140 pounds for the past 10 years. She can do most activities of daily living unassisted, but her neighbor does the grocery shopping. She verbalizes embarrassment over the effects of the aging process and stooped posture, stating that she has noticed a decrease in her height over the past year. Mrs. Clement reports frequent low back aches with occasional sharp pains. She tries to avoid bending to prevent pain, uses a heating pad, and takes Tylenol two or three times a day, which temporarily relieves the pain. She experienced menopause at the age of 50 years and has never used estrogen replacement therapy.

Physical examination reveals her to be 5 feet 2 inches tall. Two years ago, her height was 5 feet 3 1/2 inches. Her gait is wide-based and slow. Her temporomandibular joint (TMJ) has full range of motion (ROM) against resistance. She has apparent kyphosis of the cervical spine. Her paravertebrals are tender to palpation. Lower back pain is aggravated by ROM, is limited to the lower lumbar area, and does not radiate down the leg. The result of Lasègue's test is negative. No leg redness, nodules, tenderness, or swelling can be observed. The ROM of the cervical spine and upper extremities are within normal range against gravity but decreased against resistance. Lumbar flexion is 50 degrees; lateral bending is 25 degrees. The legs are equal in length. The shoulders, elbows, wrists, and fingers are symmetric, without redness, heat, swelling, or nodules. Some muscle atrophy is apparent in the upper extremities. The results of Phalen's test and Tinel's test are positive. The hips, knees, ankles, and toes are symmetric, without redness, swelling, heat, or nodules. The lower extremities have full ROM against gravity but decreased ROM against resistance.

■ Chapter Post-test

Choose the one best answer for each of the following multiple-choice questions.

_____ 1. A client visits the clinic and tells the nurse that she has joint pain in her hands, especially in the morning. The nurse should assess the client further for signs and symptoms of

 A. arthritis.

 B. osteoporosis.

 C. carpal tunnel syndrome.

 D. a neurologic disorder.

_____ 2. A client with insulin-dependent diabetes visits the clinic and complains of painful hip joints. The nurse should assess the client carefully for signs and symptoms of

   A. arthritis.

   B. gait difficulties.

   C. osteomyelitis.

   D. scoliosis.

_____ 3. A female client visits the clinic and tells the nurse that she began menarche at the age of 16 years. The nurse should instruct the client that she is at a higher risk for

   A. osteoporosis.

   B. osteomyelitis.

   C. rheumatoid arthritis.

   D. lordosis.

_____ 4. The nurse is planning a presentation on osteoporosis to a group of high school students. Which of the following should the nurse plan to include in the presentation?

   A. Bone density rises to a peak at age 50 for both sexes.

   B. Bone density in the Asian population is higher than in the white population.

   C. Moderate strenuous exercise tends to increase bone density.

   D. Approximately 5 million fractures in the United States are due to osteoporosis.

_____ 5. The nurse is caring for an adult client who is in a cast because of a fractured arm. To promote healing of the bone and tissue, the nurse should instruct the client to eat a diet that is high in

   A. whole grains.

   B. vitamin B.

   C. vitamin E.

   D. vitamin C.

_____ 6. An adult client tells the nurse that he eats sardines every day. The nurse should instruct the client that a diet high in purines can contribute to

   A. gouty arthritis.

   B. osteomalacia.

   C. bone fractures.

   D. osteomyelitis.

_____ 7. A client tells the nurse that his grandmother had a diagnosis of osteomalacia. The nurse should instruct the client that to decrease the risk factors for osteomalacia, the client should have adequate amounts of

   A. vitamin E.

   B. riboflavin.

   C. beta-carotene.

   D. vitamin D.

_____ 8. The nurse is preparing to perform a musculoskeletal examination on an adult client. The nurse has explained the examination procedure to the client. The nurse determines that the client needs **further** instructions when the client says

A. "You will be asking me to change positions often."

B. "You'll be comparing bilateral joints."

C. "You'll be assessing the size and strength of my joints."

D. "You'll continue with range of motion even if I have discomfort."

_____ 9. While assessing muscle strength in an older adult client, the nurse determines that the client's knee joint has a rating of 3 and exhibits active motion against gravity. The nurse should document the client's muscle strength as being/having

A. normal.

B. slight weakness.

C. average weakness.

D. poor range of motion.

_____ 10. While assessing an adult client's jaw, the nurse hears a clicking, popping sound, and the client expresses pain in the joint. The nurse should further assess the client for

A. arthritis.

B. TMJ dysfunction.

C. bruxism.

D. previous fracture.

_____ 11. While examining the spine of an adult client, the nurse notes that the client has a flattened lumbar curvature. The nurse should refer the client to a physician for possible

A. herniated disc.

B. scoliosis.

C. kyphosis.

D. cervical disc degeneration.

_____ 12. The nurse is assessing the spine of an adult client and detects lateral curvature of the thoracic spine with an increase in convexity on the left curved side. The nurse suspects that the client is experiencing

A. lordosis.

B. arthritis.

C. kyphosis.

D. scoliosis.

_____ 13. A client visits the clinic and tells the nurse that he has had lower back pain for the past several days. To perform Lasègue's test, the nurse should ask the client to

A. bend backward toward the nurse.

B. lean forward and touch his toes.

C. twist the shoulders in both directions.

D. lie flat and raise his leg to the point of pain.

_____ 14. An older adult client visits the clinic and tells the nurse that she has had shooting pains in both of her legs. The nurse should assess the client for signs and symptoms of

   A. herniated intervertebral disc.

   B. rheumatoid arthritis.

   C. osteoporosis.

   D. metastases.

_____ 15. While assessing the range of motion in an adult client's shoulders, the client expresses pain and exhibits limited abduction and muscle weakness. The nurse plans to refer the client to a physician for possible

   A. rotator cuff tear.

   B. nerve damage.

   C. cervical disc degeneration.

   D. tendonitis.

_____ 16. While assessing an older adult client, the client complains of chronic pain and severe limitation of all shoulder movements. The nurse should refer the client to a physician for possible

   A. rotator cuff tendonitis.

   B. rheumatoid arthritis.

   C. calcified tendinitis.

   D. chronic bursitis.

_____ 17. The nurse is examining an adult client's range of motion in the shoulders. The client is unable to shrug her shoulders against resistance. The nurse suspects that the client has a lesion of cranial nerve

   A. VIII.

   B. IX.

   C. X.

   D. XI.

_____ 18. While assessing the elbow of an adult client, the client complains of pain and swelling. The nurse should further assess the client for

   A. arthritis.

   B. ganglion cyst.

   C. carpal tunnel syndrome.

   D. nerve damage.

_____ 19. While reviewing a client's chart before seeing the client for the first time, the nurse notes that the client has a diagnosis of Dupuytren's contracture. The nurse anticipates that the client will exhibit

   A. inability to turn the wrists.

   B. ulnar deviation of the hands.

   C. flexion of the distal interphalangeal joints.

   D. inability to extend the ring and little finger.

_____ 20. While assessing the musculoskeletal system of an adult client, the nurse observes hard, painless nodules over the distal interphalangeal joints. The nurse should document the presence of

A. osteoarthritis.

B. bursitis.

C. tendonitis.

D. rheumatoid arthritis.

_____ 21. A client visits the clinic and complains of wrist pain. To perform Phalen's test, the nurse should ask the client to

A. move the hand inward with the wrists straight.

B. place both palms on the examination table.

C. flex both wrists against resistance.

D. place the backs of both hands against each other.

_____ 22. While assessing an adult client, the nurse tests the client for Tinel's sign. The nurse should instruct the client that numbness or tingling may indicate

A. arthritis.

B. carpal tunnel syndrome.

C. tenosynovitis.

D. crepitus.

_____ 23. While assessing the musculoskeletal system of an adult client, the nurse detects tenderness, warmth, and a boggy consistency of the client's knee. The nurse should refer the client to a physician for possible

A. torn meniscus.

B. malignancy.

C. fracture.

D. synovitis.

_____ 24. A client visits the clinic and complains of pain in his knees. The nurse explains that a ballottement test will be performed. To perform the ballottement test, the nurse should

A. place the left thumb and index finger on either side of the patella.

B. use the ball of the hand to firmly stroke the medial side of the knee.

C. press the lateral side of the knee and inspect for swelling.

D. palpate for tenderness 10 centimeters above the patella.

_____ 25. While assessing an older adult client, the nurse notes decreased range of motion and crepitation as the client tries to bend his knees to his chest. The nurse determines that the client is most likely experiencing

A. flexion contractures.

B. signs of aging.

C. osteoarthritis.

D. genu valgum.

_____ 26. A client visits the clinic and tells the nurse that after playing softball yesterday, he thinks his knee is "locking up." The nurse should perform the McMurray's test by asking the client to

   A. move from a standing to a squatting position.

   B. raise his leg while in a supine position.

   C. bend forward while trying to touch the toes.

   D. flex the knee and hip while in a supine position.

_____ 27. While assessing the feet of an adult client, the nurse notes that the client's great toes are deviated, with overlapping of the second toes. The client states that there is pain on the medial side. The nurse should refer the client to a physician for possible

   A. hallux valgus.

   B. pes planus.

   C. pes cavus.

   D. verruca vulgaris.

_____ 28. While reviewing a client's chart before seeing the client for the first time, the nurse notes that the client has a diagnosis of pes planus. The nurse anticipates that the client has

   A. high arches.

   B. bunions.

   C. calluses.

   D. flat feet.

_____ 29. While assessing the feet of an older adult client, the nurse observes that the metatarsophalangeal joint of the client's great toe is tender, reddened, and painful. The nurse should refer the client to a physician for possible

   A. bunions.

   B. corns.

   C. hammer toe.

   D. gouty arthritis.

_____ 30. While assessing the feet of an adult client, the nurse observes hyperextension of the metatarsophalangeal joint. with flexion at the proximal interphalangeal joint on the client's second toes. The nurse should refer the client to a physician for possible

   A. hammer toes.

   B. gouty arthritis.

   C. calluses.

   D. hallux valgus.

_____ 31. While assessing the feet of an adult client, the nurse observes tiny dark spots under a painful callus on the client's foot. The nurse should document the presence of

   A. corns.

   B. bunions.

   C. plantar warts.

   D. gouty arthritis.

CROSSWORD PUZZLE

Complete the following crossword puzzle to become more familiar with the terminology used with assessment of the musculoskeletal system.

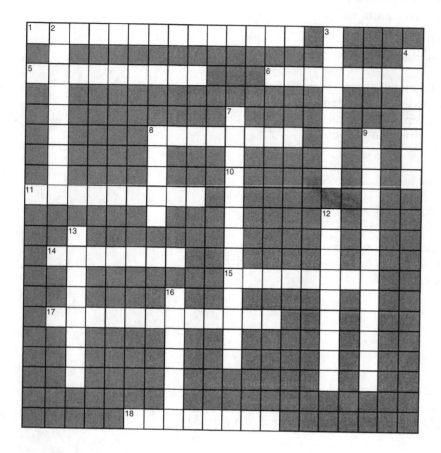

ACROSS

1. Goniometer is used to measure this-also phrase used to describe joint capability
5. Movement of the limbs or the trunk and head toward the median plane of the body
6. Outward turning of a limb: ___ rotation
8. Inflammation of a bursa
10. Spasmodic alternation of muscular contraction and relaxation
11. Fixation of a joint, often in an abnormal position; seen frequently with rheumatoid arthritis
14. Tenderness or pain in the muscle
15. Type of rigidity characterized by jerky movements when the muscle is passively stretched
17. Backward bending or flexion of a joint
18. Abnormal anterior concavity of the spine

DOWN

2. Movement of the limbs or the trunk and head, away from the median plane of the body
3. Dry, crackling sound or sensation heard or felt as a joint is moved through its ROM
4. Movement that brings a limb into or toward a bent condition
7. Circular movement of a limb
8. A fibrous fluid-filled sac found between certain tendons and the bones beneath them
9. The localized, uncoordinated twitching of a single muscle group
12. Movement that brings a limb into or toward a straight condition
13. Abnormal convexity of the posterior curve of the spine
16. Type of flexion associated with extension of the foot

■ Self-Reflection and Evaluation
of Learner Objectives

After you have read Chapter 22 and completed the above quizzes and activities, please identify to what degree you have met each of the following chapter learning objectives. For those objectives that you have met partially or not at all, you will want to review chapter content for that learning objective.

Objective	Very much	Somewhat	Not at all
1. Describe the structure and functions of the bones, skeletal muscles, and joints.			
2. Discuss risk factors for osteoporosis and ways to reduce these risk factors.			
3. Discuss the incidence of osteoporosis across cultures.			
4. Obtain an accurate nursing history of the client's muscles, joints, and bones.			
5. Explain how to prepare the client for an examination of the muscles, joints, and bones.			
6. Describe the equipment necessary to perform a musculoskeletal assessment.			
7. Describe the two physical examination techniques (inspection and palpation) used to complete a musculoskeletal assessment.			
8. Assess the client's gait.			
9. Assess the client's joints for position, ROM, suppleness of movement, swelling, redness, tenderness or pain, bony overgrowths, alignment with other joints and bones, and associated muscle development and muscle strength.			
10. Perform test for carpal tunnel syndrome.			
11. Describe expected aging changes of the musculoskeletal system.			

For additional information on this book, be sure to visit *http://connection.lww.com.*

CHAPTER 23

Neurologic Assessment

CHAPTER OVERVIEW

Just as the musculoskeletal system structures the body, so the neurologic system structures thought, movement and balance, sensation, and communication, among other life functions. Quality of life is significantly affected by the health of the neurologic system.

■ Chapter Pretest

MULTIPLE CHOICE

Choose the one best answer for each of the following multiple-choice questions.

_____ 1. The cerebrospinal fluid cushions the central nervous system (CNS), provides nourishment to the CNS, and

    A. transmits impulses.

    B. coats the brain.

    C. regulates heart rate.

    D. removes wastes.

_____ 2. The cerebrum is divided into right and left hemispheres, which are joined together by the

    A. corpus callosum.

    B. diencephalon.

    C. medulla oblongata.

    D. pons.

_____ 3. The portion of the brain that rims the surfaces of the cerebral hemispheres forming the cerebral cortex is the

    A. gray matter.

    B. cerebellum.

    C. diencephalon.

    D. brainstem.

_____ 4. The diencephalon of the brain consists of the

    A. pons and brainstem.

    B. medulla oblongata and cerebrum.

    C. cerebellum and midbrain.

    D. thalamus and hypothalamus.

_____ 5. The hypothalamus is responsible for regulating

    A. sleep cycles.

    B. nerve impulses.

    C. memory.

    D. eye reflexes.

MATCHING

Match the terms in the left column with the correct descriptions in the right column.

Term	Description
_____ 1. Spinal accessory	A. Carries sensations from the throat, larynx, heart, lungs, bronchi, gastrointestinal tract, and abdominal viscera
_____ 2. Glossopharyngeal	B. Innervates neck muscles that promote movement of the shoulders and head rotation
_____ 3. Olfactory	C. Carries visual impulses from the eye to the brain
_____ 4. Facial	D. Contracts eye muscles to control eye movement, constricts pupils, and elevates eyelids
_____ 5. Hypoglossal	E. Contains sensory fibers for taste on posterior one third of the tongue; responsible for "gag reflex" when stimulated
_____ 6. Acoustic	F. Contracts one eye muscle to control inferomedial eye movement
_____ 7. Optic	G. Innervates tongue muscles that promote the movement of food and talking
_____ 8. Vagus	H. Carries smell impulses from nasal mucous membrane to brain
_____ 9. Abducens	I. Carries sensory impulses of pain, touch, and temperature from the face to the brain
_____ 10. Oculomotor	J. Controls lateral eye movements
_____ 11. Trigeminal	K. Contains sensory fibers for hearing and balance
_____ 12. Trochlear	L. Contains sensory fibers for taste on anterior two thirds of the tongue, and stimulates secretions from the salivary glands and tears from lacrimal glands

LABELING ACTIVITY

Label the structures of the brain.

Structures of the brain.

Label the structure indicated by the line; then match your answer with the label on the matching figure in chapter 23 of your textbook.

Label this cross-section of the spinal cord.

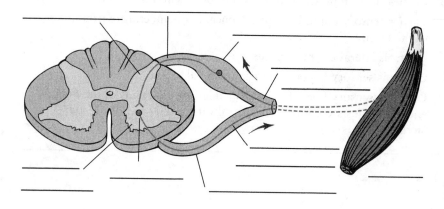

Cross-section of spinal cord.

Label the structure indicated by the line; then match your answer with the label on the matching figure in chapter 23 of your textbook.

■ Learner Activities

After reading Chapter 23, participate in the following learning activities.

WORKING WITH PEERS IN LEARNING LAB

1. With a lab partner, label the 12 cranial nerves on the diagram below. After completing the labels, assess the function of each nerve on each of the others.

Twelve cranial nerves emerging from brain.

Label the structure indicated by the line; then match your answer with the label on the matching figure in chapter 23 of your textbook.

2. Refer to the Risk Factors box in Chapter 23. Then assess a lab partner's risk for cerebrovascular accident (CVA, stroke).

3. Practice testing balance safely with a lab partner.

INTERVIEWING AND RECORDING ASSESSMENT FINDINGS

Use the following Nursing History Checklist as your guide to interviewing and recording the findings from a neurologic assessment.

NURSING HISTORY CHECKLIST

Questions	Normal findings	Abnormal findings	Additional data needed
Current Symptoms			
1. Headaches, numbness, or tingling?			
2. Seizure activity?			
3. Dizziness, lightheadedness, or problems with balance or coordination?			
4. Decrease in ability to smell or taste?			
5. Ringing in ears?			
6. Change in vision?			
7. Difficulty understanding when people are talking to you or when you talk to others?			
8. Difficulty swallowing?			
9. Loss of bowel or bladder control?			
10. Memory loss?			
11. Tremors?			

(continues)

NURSING HISTORY CHECKLIST *(Continued)*

Questions	Normal findings	Abnormal findings	Additional data needed
Past History			
1. Head injury?			
2. Meningitis?			
3. Encephalitis?			
4. Spinal cord injury?			
5. Stroke?			
6. Treatment received?			
Family History			
1. High blood pressure?			
2. Stroke?			
3. Alzheimer's disease?			
4. Epilepsy?			
5. Brain cancer?			
6. Huntington's chorea?			
Lifestyle and Health Practices			
1. Any prescription or nonprescription medications?			
2. Smoking?			
3. Wearing of seat belts/protective head gear?			
4. Daily diet?			
5. Exposure to lead, insecticides, pollutants, chemicals?			
6. Lifting of heavy objects?			
7. Frequent repetitive movements?			
8. Functioning/daily activities?			
Reflexes			
1. Test deep tendon reflexes.			
2. Test superficial reflexes.			
3. Test for meningeal irritation/inflammation (if indicated).			
Analysis of Data			
1. Formulate nursing diagnoses (wellness, risk, actual).			
2. Formulate collaborative problems.			
3. Make necessary referrals.			

PERFORMING PHYSICAL ASSESSMENT

Use the following Physical Assessment Checklist as your guide to performing a neurologic assessment.

PHYSICAL ASSESSMENT CHECKLIST

Assessment Skill	Findings (Normal or Abnormal) and Notes		Performance (Satisfactory, Needs Improvement, Unsatisfactory)		
	N	**A**	**S**	**N**	**U**
1. Gather equipment, such as examination gloves, Mini-Mental State Examination, pencil and paper, cotton-tipped applicators, newsprint to read, ophthalmoscope, paper clip, penlight, Snellen chart, sterile cotton ball, substances to smell and taste, tongue blade, tuning fork, tape measure, cotton balls, objects to feel, test tubes with hot and cold water, tuning fork (low-pitched), and reflex hammer.	☐	☐	☐	☐	☐
2. Explain procedure to client, and ask client to put on a gown.	☐	☐	☐	☐	☐
Mental Status					
1. Assess level of consciousness.	☐	☐	☐	☐	☐
2. Observe appearance and behavior.	☐	☐	☐	☐	☐
3. Observe mood, feelings, and expressions.	☐	☐	☐	☐	☐
4. Observe thought processes and perceptions.	☐	☐	☐	☐	☐
5. Observe cognitive abilities.	☐	☐	☐	☐	☐
Cranial Nerves					
1. Test cranial nerve I-olfactory.	☐	☐	☐	☐	☐
2. Test cranial nerve II-optic.	☐	☐	☐	☐	☐
3. Test cranial nerve III-oculomotor.	☐	☐	☐	☐	☐
4. Test cranial nerve IV-trochlear.	☐	☐	☐	☐	☐
5. Test cranial nerve VI-abducens.	☐	☐	☐	☐	☐
6. Test cranial nerve V-trigeminal.	☐	☐	☐	☐	☐
7. Test cranial nerve VII-facial.	☐	☐	☐	☐	☐
8. Test cranial nerve VIII-acoustic (vestibulocochlear).	☐	☐	☐	☐	☐
9. Test cranial nerve IX-glossopharyngeal.	☐	☐	☐	☐	☐
10. Test cranial nerve X-vagus.	☐	☐	☐	☐	☐
11. Test cranial nerve XI-spinal accessory.	☐	☐	☐	☐	☐
12. Test cranial nerve XII-hypoglossal.	☐	☐	☐	☐	☐
Motor and Cerebellar Systems					
1. Test condition and movement of muscles.	☐	☐	☐	☐	☐
2. Test balance.	☐	☐	☐	☐	☐
3. Test coordination.	☐	☐	☐	☐	☐
4. Test light touch, pain, and temperature sensations.	☐	☐	☐	☐	☐
5. Test vibratory sensations.	☐	☐	☐	☐	☐
6. Test position sensations.	☐	☐	☐	☐	☐
7. Test tactile discrimination (fine touch).	☐	☐	☐	☐	☐

CRITICAL THINKING AND CASE STUDIES

1. Read the following case study, and then formulate wellness, risk, and actual nursing diagnoses and identify collaborative problems for the client and his wife. Also develop nursing interventions to assist this family.

Mr. R., aged 74, has had Parkinson's disease for more than 10 years. His primary caregiver is his wife of 52 years, who is in good health except for rheumatoid arthritis. The couple's grown sons live in another state but visit the family once a year during the Christmas holidays. Recently Mr. R. has experienced a greater degree of twitching in his arms. He slurs his speech and is difficult to understand at times. He and his wife had enjoyed a wide range of activities, such as bowling, going to the movies, and trying new restaurants. However, since his condition has deteriorated they rarely leave the house. Mr. R. has also experienced difficulty walking and getting up from the bed or chair. His wife must assist him in all activities of daily living.

2. On the basis of the following assessment information, work through the steps of analyzing the data. Identify abnormal data and strengths in *subjective and objective* findings, assemble *cue clusters,* draw *inferences,* make possible *nursing diagnoses,* identify *defining characteristics, confirm or rule out the nursing diagnosis,* and *document* your conclusions.

Use the blank diagnostic analysis charts provided at the end of this book to guide your thinking. You may want to write on the chart or use separate paper. Propose nursing diagnoses that are specific to the client in the case study. Identify collaborative problems, if any, for this client. Finally, identify data, if any, that point toward a medical problem requiring a referral.

Mr. Kay is a 72-year-old man who had a right hemisphere thrombotic stroke 14 days ago and was discharged to his home from the 51st State Stroke Rehabilitation Center. His primary caregiver is his 68-year-old wife, who is in good health. He has a daughter and son, who live within a 50-mile radius and visit frequently. Before the CVA, Mr. Kay was very active and independent, a retired banker who loved to golf and travel. He received a diagnosis of hypertension 15 years ago but had poor compliance in taking prescribed medications. "When my blood pressure was checked, it was normal, so why take the medicine if I don't need it!" The CVA resulted in deficits in his visual, tactile, and kinesthetic senses. He denies his disabilities and frequently displays poor judgment and impulsive behavior. Mr. Kay requires partial assistance with activities of daily living, feeding, and mobility. While in rehabilitation he seemed to learn best if given brief, simple cues. Because of visual disturbance, he has difficulty with visual cues.

When interviewed, Mr. Kay states he has weakness and numbness of his left arm and leg and that he often has to look at his left arm and leg to determine where they are. He also states that he frequently loses his balance and has occasional dizziness when getting up in the morning. He has difficulty with dressing and grooming and frequently confuses his comb with his toothbrush and puts his clothes on inside out. He is frustrated at not being able to care for himself. He has been prescribed a 2-gram-per-day sodium diet; however, he has a poor appetite. He states that the "food doesn't taste or smell good." His wife states that it often takes him a long time to complete a meal, and he frequently leaves food on the left side of the plate. When asked about changes in memory or concentration, his wife states, "Now, it's difficult for him to remember dates and phone numbers, but he knows people's names."

Your physical assessment reveals the following:

- Mental status: awake, alert, oriented to person, place, and usually time. Communicates verbally, although comprehension is questionable at times. Eye contact poor. Mood seems anxious. Dress clean, shirt is on inside out. Difficulty in recalling recent dates and events. Unable to interpret written instructions. Reads a few sentences at a time; loses place on page frequently. Unable to recognize familiar objects such as toothbrush and comb. Unable to draw left side of clock. Mini-Mental State Exam score: 21.

- Cranial nerves: intact except for cranial nerve II; loses place on page after reading a few sentences. Unable to record visual stimuli from the left side because of homonymous hemianopsia.

- Motor and cerebellar systems: gait slow and unsteady with one person assisting; abnormal tandem walk. Muscle strength weak in left upper and lower extremities. Unable to assess finger coordination and fine motor function of left upper and lower extremities.

- Sensory system: decreased light, sharp, dull touch; vibratory, two-point sensation in left upper and lower extremity; unable to identify safety pin and number traced on palm of left hand.

- Reflexes: 1+ left upper and lower extremities; 2+ right upper and lower extremities; down-going toes with plantar stimulation.

■ Chapter Post-test

MULTIPLE CHOICE QUESTIONS

Choose the one best answer for each of the following multiple-choice questions.

_____ 1. Sensations of temperature, pain, and crude and light touch are carried by way of the
   A. extrapyramidal tract.
   B. corticospinal tract.
   C. spinothalamic tract.
   D. posterior tract.

_____ 2. The cranial nerve that has sensory fibers for taste and fibers that result in the "gag reflex" is the
   A. vagus.
   B. hypoglossal.
   C. trigeminal.
   D. glossopharyngeal.

_____ 3. The nurse is assessing an older adult client when the client tells the nurse that she has experienced transient blind spots for the last few days. The nurse should refer the client to a physician for possible

A. vagus nerve damage.

B. cerebral vascular accident.

C. spinal cord compression.

D. Parkinson's disease.

_____ 4. The nurse is planning a presentation to a group of adults on the topic of cardiovascular accidents. Which of the following should the nurse plan to include in the teaching plan?

A. Strokes are the number one cause of death in the United States.

B. Smoking and high cholesterol levels are risk factors for CVA.

C. Clients who smoke while taking oral contraceptives are not at higher risk.

D. Postmenopausal women taking estrogen are at greater risk for CVA.

_____ 5. The nurse is caring for a client during the immediate postoperative period after abdominal surgery. While performing a "neuro check" the nurse should assess the client's

A. sensation in the extremities.

B. deep tendon reflexes.

C. ability to speak.

D. recent memory.

_____ 6. The nurse is preparing to percuss a client's reflexes in his arms. To use the reinforcement technique, the nurse should ask the client to

A. clench his jaw.

B. stretch the opposite arm.

C. hold his neck toward the floor.

D. straighten his legs forward.

_____ 7. The Glasgow Coma Scale measures the level of consciousness in clients who are at high risk for rapid deterioration of the nervous system. A score of 13 indicates

A. deep coma.

B. severe impairment.

C. no verbal response.

D. some impairment.

_____ 8. A client visits the clinic and tells the nurse that he has not been feeling very well. The nurse observes that the client's speech is slow, the client has a disheveled appearance, and he maintains poor eye contact with the nurse. The nurse should further assess the client for

A. depression.

B. delirium.

C. hallucinations.

D. schizophrenia.

_____ 9. While assessing the neurologic system of a confused older adult, the nurse observes that the client is unable to recall past events. The nurse suspects that the client may be exhibiting signs of

A. depression.

B. anxiety.

C. attention deficit disorder.

D. cerebral cortex disorder.

_____ 10. The nurse is assessing the neurologic system of an adult client. To test the client's use of memory to learn new information, the nurse should ask the client

A. "What did you have for breakfast?"

B. "How old were you when you began working?"

C. "Can you repeat _rose, hose, nose, clothes_?"

D. "Can you repeat _brown, chair, textbook, tomato_?"

_____ 11. While assessing the pupils of a hospitalized adult client, the nurse observes that the client's pupils are dilated to 6 centimeters. The nurse suspects that the client is exhibiting signs of

A. oculomotor nerve paralysis.

B. damage to the pons.

C. alcohol abuse.

D. cocaine abuse.

_____ 12. The nurse is assessing the neurologic system of an adult client. To test the client's motor function of the facial nerve, the nurse should

A. ask the client to purse the lips.

B. ask the client to open the mouth and say "ah."

C. note the presence of a gag reflex.

D. observe the client swallow a sip of water.

_____ 13. The nurse is assessing the neurologic system of a client who has spastic muscle tone. The nurse should explain to the client that spastic muscle tone is associated with impairment to the

A. extrapyramidal tract.

B. spinothalamic tract.

C. posterior columns.

D. corticospinal tract.

_____ 14. The nurse is preparing to perform the Romberg test on an adult male client. The nurse should instruct the client to

A. squat down as far as he is able to do so.

B. keep his eyes open while he bends at the knees.

C. stand erect with arms at the sides and feet together.

D. touch the tip of his nose with his finger.

_____ 15. The nurse is planning to test position sensation in an adult female client. To perform this procedure, the nurse should ask the client to close her eyes while the nurse moves the client's

    A. arm away from the body.

    B. toes up or down.

    C. hand forward and then backward.

    D. leg away from the body.

_____ 16. While assessing the Achilles reflex in an 84-year-old client, the nurse observes that the Achilles reflex is difficult to elicit. The nurse should

    A. refer the client to a physician for further evaluation.

    B. ask the client about injuries to the feet.

    C. determine whether the client is having any pain in the feet.

    D. document the finding in the client's record.

_____ 17. While assessing the plantar reflex of an adult client, the nurse observes a positive Babinski reflex. The nurse suspects that the client may be exhibiting signs of

    A. meningeal irritation.

    B. diabetes mellitus.

    C. drug intoxication.

    D. lower motor neuron lesions.

■ Self-Reflection and Evaluation of Learner Objectives

After you have read Chapter 23 and completed the above quizzes and activities, please identify to what degree you have met each of the following chapter learning objectives. For those objectives that you have met partially or not at all, you will want to review chapter content for that learning objective.

Objective	Very much	Somewhat	Not at all
1. Describe the structures and function of the central and peripheral nervous system.			
2. Identify the 12 cranial nerves and name their functions.			
3. Obtain an accurate nursing history of a client's neurologic system.			
4. Identify the five major areas involved in a complete neurologic examination.			
5. Explain how to prepare a client for a neurologic examination.			
6. Describe the equipment necessary for examining the neurologic system.			
7. Assess the client's level of consciousness and orientation.			

Objective	Very much	Somewhat	Not at all
8. Assess the client's appearance and behavior, including posture, body movements, grooming, hygiene, facial expressions, speech, mood, and feelings.			
9. Assess length of concentration in an adult client.			
10. Assess recent and remote memory of an adult client. Also assess the client's use of memory to learn new information.			
11. Assess abstract reasoning ability, judgment, and visual, perceptual, and constructional ability of an adult client.			
12. Assess the client using the Mini-mental State Examination.			
13. Assess cranial nerve function of an adult client.			
14. Assess the condition and movement of all muscle groups of the client. Also assess balance and coordination.			
15. Assess light touch, pain, and temperature sensation of an adult.			
16. Assess vibratory sensation, position sensation, and fine touch (tactile discrimination) of the client.			
17. Assess deep tendon reflexes and then superficial reflexes of an adult client.			
18. Assess the client for meningeal irritation.			
19. Identify and discuss nursing diagnoses and collaborative problems for clients experiencing abnormalities of the neurologic system.			

For additional information on this book, be sure to visit *http://connection.lww.com.*

UNIT III

Nursing Assessment of Special Groups

CHAPTER 24

Assessment of Infants, Children, and Adolescents

CHAPTER OVERVIEW

Over about 18 years, the human being progresses from infancy to adulthood. Rapid physical and mental growth and development occur in many stages, during which health care is particularly important in preventing and detecting disorders and abnormalities that may inhibit growth and retard the fulfillment of potential. Nursing assessment plays a key role in supporting the health of growing young people.

■ Chapter Pretest

MULTIPLE CHOICE

Choose the one best answer for each of the following multiple-choice questions.

_____ 1. While assessing the skin, hair, and nails of a 4-year-old boy, the nurse can anticipate that the child will have
   A. functioning apocrine glands.
   B. a thin layer of subcutaneous fat.
   C. fine downy hairs on his body.
   D. smooth-textured skin.

_____ 2. The anterior fontanelle of a neonate closes between
   A. 2 and 3 months.
   B. 4 and 6 months.
   C. 7 and 11 months.
   D. 12 and 18 months.

_____ 3. The nurse is planning a presentation on childhood growth and development to a group of new parents. Which of the following should the nurse include in the teaching plan?
   A. A child's head reaches 90% of its full growth by 6 years of age.
   B. Half of a child's postnatal brain growth is achieved by 3 years of age.
   C. During the school-age years, the cranium grows faster than the face.
   D. Lymphoid tissue reaches adult size by 4 years of age.

_____ 4. The nurse is planning to instruct a first-time mother about her new-born. The nurse should plan to instruct the mother that the newborn
   A. is an obligatory nose breather.
   B. will have deciduous teeth by 3 months.
   C. who drools is preparing for tooth eruption.
   D. will develop permanent teeth in the jaw by 6 years of age.

_____ 5. The nurse is preparing to assess the heart sounds in a 3-year-old child. To locate the apical impulse, the nurse should plan to place the stethoscope at the child's
   A. second intercostal space.
   B. third intercostal space.
   C. fourth intercostal space.
   D. fifth intercostal space.

MATCHING

Match the following descriptions with the appropriate age group.

Term	Description	
_____ 1.	Engages in parallel play	A. Infants
_____ 2.	Likes explanations and demonstrations in health teaching	B. Toddlers
_____ 3.	Peak age group for separation anxiety	C. Preschoolers
_____ 4.	Confidentiality a must	D. School-agers
_____ 5.	Gains 15 to 65 pounds during this stage	E. Adolescents
_____ 6.	Bow-leggedness is typical	
_____ 7.	Girls surpass boys in growth during this period	
_____ 8.	Weight triples during this period	
_____ 9.	Pincer grasp develops	
_____ 10.	Visual capacity reaches adult level of 20/20	
_____ 11.	Sensorimotor stage is completed in this period	
_____ 12.	Ability to listen and comprehend starts during this stage	
_____ 13.	Vocabulary ranges from 900 to 2100 words	
_____ 14.	Develops ability to think beyond the present	
_____ 15.	Has ability to decide between two socially accepted standards	
_____ 16.	Must have needs met consistently to develop sense of trust	
_____ 17.	The age of "magical thinking"	
_____ 18.	Learns rules and competition	
_____ 19.	Develops lifelong eating patterns	
_____ 20.	Should sleep in supine position to minimize risk of sudden infant death syndrome (SIDS)	

■ Learner Activities

After reading Chapter 24 participate in the following learning activities.

1. Describe how you would perform the following:
   a. an otoscopic examination on a feisty 2-year-old
   b. abdominal palpation on a ticklish 9-year-old
   c. the patellar reflex on a 4-year-old who kicks before you strike
   d. the psychosocial history of a 16-year-old

WORKING WITH PEERS IN LEARNING LAB

Discuss with a lab partner how you would handle the following situations.

1. While performing an assessment of a 15-year-old girl, you note that she is quiet and withdrawn. She complains of multiple vague physical complaints and gives you her favorite watch, stating, "I know you'll take real good care of this." Discuss what you would do next.

2. A 4-month-old is brought in for well child care. The mother asks, "What is my baby going to have done today?" Using the American Academy of Pediatrics' recommendations for well child care, describe what you would include in your reply.

3. You are going to give a 30-minute talk to a PTA group on the health needs of school-aged children. Considering that you are addressing a group whose children's ages range from 6 to 12 years, discuss what you would include in your talk.

INTERVIEWING AND RECORDING ASSESSMENT FINDINGS

Use the following Nursing History Checklist as your guide to interviewing and recording the findings of a pediatric assessment.

NURSING HISTORY CHECKLIST

Questions	Normal findings	Abnormal findings	Additional data needed
Current Symptoms			
1. Child's reason for seeking health care or the parent's (informant's) reason for seeking health care for the child?			
Current Health/Illness Status			
1. Symptom analysis of chief complaint?			
2. Other current or recurrent illnesses or problems?			
3. Any other health concerns?			
4. Current medication used?			

(continues)

NURSING HISTORY CHECKLIST *(Continued)*

Questions	Normal findings	Abnormal findings	Additional data needed

Past History

1. Birth history (pregnancy, labor and delivery, perinatal history)?

2. Previous illnesses, injuries, or surgeries?

3. Allergies (and reactions to same)?

4. Immunization status?

5. Growth and developmental milestones?

6. Habits?

Review of Systems

1. General: overall health status?

2. Integument: lesions, bruising, care habits?

3. Head: trauma, headaches?

4. Eyes: visual acuity, last eye exam, drainage, infections?

5. Ears: hearing acuity, last hearing exam, drainage, infections?

6. Nose: bleeding, congestion, discharge?

7. Mouth: lesions, soreness, tooth eruption, patterns of dental care, last dental exam?

8. Throat: sore throat frequency, hoarseness, difficulty swallowing?

9. Neck: stiffness, tenderness?

10. Chest: pain, cough, wheezing, shortness of breath, asthma, infections?

11. Breasts: thelarche, lesions, discharge, performance of breast self-examination (BSE)?

12. Cardiovascular: history of murmurs, exercise tolerance, dizziness, palpitations, congenital defects?

13. Gastrointestinal: appetite, bowel habits, food intolerances, nausea, vomiting, pain, history of parasites?

14. Genitourinary: urgency, frequency, discharge, urinary tract infections, sexually transmitted diseases, enuresis, sexual problems or dysfunctions (male), performance of testicular self-examination?

15. Gynecologic: menarche, menstrual history, sexual problems or dysfunctions?

16. Musculoskeletal: pain, swelling, fractures, mobility problems, scoliosis?

17. Neurologic: ataxia, tremors, unusual movements, seizures?

18. Lymphatic: pain, swelling or tenderness, enlargement of spleen or liver?

(continues)

NURSING HISTORY CHECKLIST *(Continued)*

Questions	Normal findings	Abnormal findings	Additional data needed
19. Endocrine/metabolic: growth patterns, polyuria, polydypsia, polyphagia?			
20. Psychiatric history: any psychiatric, developmental, substance abuse, or eating disorder?			

Family History

1. Family genetic traits or diseases with familial tendencies?

2. Communicable diseases?

3. Psychiatric disorders?

4. Substance abuse?

Nutritional History

1. Determine the quantity and the types of food or formula ingested daily: use 24-hour recall, food diary for 3 days (2 weekdays and 1 weekend day), or food frequency record.

2. Ask if child has any problem with feeding.

3. Ask if child uses any vitamin supplements.

4. Ask if child is on special diet.

5. Ask if there are any cultural or religious preferences.

6. Assess dieting behaviors: include body image, types of diets, frequency of weighing, and use of self-induced vomiting, laxatives, and diuretics.

Sleep History

1. Time child goes to bed and awakens?

2. Quality of sleep?

3. Nap history?

4. Sleep aids (blanket, toy)?

Psychosocial History

1. Home: composition of family members, occupation/education of members, culture and religion, communication patterns, family roles and relationships, financial status?

2. School: grades, behavior, relationship with teachers and peers?

3. Activities: types of play, number of hours of TV viewing per day, amount of non-school-related reading, hobbies?

4. Discipline: type and frequency used at home?

5. Sex: child's/adolescent's concerns, abuse history, sexual activity patterns, number of part-

(continues)

NURSING HISTORY CHECKLIST *(Continued)*

Questions	Normal findings	Abnormal findings	Additional data needed
ners, use of condoms and contraceptives, AIDS awareness?			
6. Substance use: amount, frequency, and circumstances of use for tobacco, alcohol, licit and illicit drugs, steroids, and substances such as inhalants?			
7. Violence: domestic violence, self-abusive behaviors, suicide ideation and attempts, violence perpetrated on others by child/adolescent being interviewed?			

Developmental Assessment

1. Assess developmental milestones in
    a. gross motor skills
    b. fine motor skills
    c. language development
    d. cognitive development
    e. social and affective development
2. Observe the child's behavior before structured interaction for spontaneous activity; observe the child's responses to the environment.
3. Administer developmental tests as appropriate for age (Denver Developmental Screening Test, Brazelton Neonatal Behavior Assessment Scale, Goodeneough-Harris Draw-A-Person Test, temperament questionnaires).

PERFORMING PHYSICAL ASSESSMENT

Use the following Physical Assessment Checklist as your guide to performing a pediatric assessment examination.

PHYSICAL ASSESSMENT CHECKLIST

Assessment Skill	Findings (Normal or Abnormal) and Notes		Performance (Satisfactory, Needs Improvement, Unsatisfactory)		
	N	A	S	N	U
1. Uses general principles:					
a. In most cases, physical assessment involves a head-to-toe examination that covers each body system.	☐	☐	☐	☐	☐
b. Complete less threatening and least intrusive procedures first, to secure child's trust.	☐	☐	☐	☐	☐
c. Explain what you will be doing and what the child can expect to feel; allow the child to manipulate equipment before it is used.	☐	☐	☐	☐	☐

PHYSICAL ASSESSMENT CHECKLIST

Assessment Skill	Findings (Normal or Abnormal) and Notes		Performance (Satisfactory, Needs Improvement, Unsatisfactory)		
	N	A	S	N	U
2. Uses developmental approaches:	☐	☐	☐	☐	☐
a. Infants: Allow infant to sit in parent's lap, encourage parents to hold infant, use distraction, enlist parent's assistance.	☐	☐	☐	☐	☐
b. Toddlers: Allow to sit on parent's lap, enlist parent's aid, use play, praise cooperation.	☐	☐	☐	☐	☐
c. Preschoolers: Use story telling, use doll and puppet play, give choices when able.	☐	☐	☐	☐	☐
d. School-age: Maintain privacy, use gown, explain procedures and equipment, teach about their bodies.	☐	☐	☐	☐	☐
e. Adolescents: Provide privacy and confidentiality, provide option of having parent present or not, emphasize normality, provide health teaching.	☐	☐	☐	☐	☐
General Appearance					
1. Inspect physical appearance.	☐	☐	☐	☐	☐
2. Assess nutritional state.	☐	☐	☐	☐	☐
3. Assess hygiene.	☐	☐	☐	☐	☐
4. Assess behavior.	☐	☐	☐	☐	☐
5. Assess interactions with parents and nurse.	☐	☐	☐	☐	☐
6. Assess overall development and speech.	☐	☐	☐	☐	☐
Vital Signs					
1. Measure blood pressure	☐	☐	☐	☐	☐
2. Measure pulse rate.	☐	☐	☐	☐	☐
3. Measure respirations.	☐	☐	☐	☐	☐
4. Measure temperature.	☐	☐	☐	☐	☐
5. Measure height and weight.	☐	☐	☐	☐	☐
6. Measure head circumference in infants.	☐	☐	☐	☐	☐
Skin, Hair, and Nails					
1. Inspect and palpate skin.					
2. Inspect and palpate hair (distribution characteristics).	☐	☐	☐	☐	☐
3. Inspect and palpate nails (texture, shape, color, condition).	☐	☐	☐	☐	☐
Head, Neck, and Cervical Lymph Nodes					
1. Inspect and palpate the head (symmetry, condition of fontanelles).	☐	☐	☐	☐	☐
2. Inspect and palpate the face.	☐	☐	☐	☐	☐
3. Inspect and palpate the neck (suppleness, lymph nodes for swelling, mobility, temperature, and tenderness).	☐	☐	☐	☐	☐

(continues)

PHYSICAL ASSESSMENT CHECKLIST

Assessment Skill	Findings (Normal or Abnormal) and Notes		Performance (Satisfactory, Needs Improvement, Unsatisfactory)		
	N	A	S	N	U
Mouth, Throat, Nose, and Sinuses					
1. Inspect mouth and throat (tooth eruption, condition of gums, lips, teeth, palpates, tonsils, tongue, buccal mucosa).	☐	☐	☐	☐	☐
2. Inspect nose and sinuses (discharge, tenderness, turbinates [color, swelling]).	☐	☐	☐	☐	☐
Eyes					
1. Inspect external eye.	☐	☐	☐	☐	☐
2. Perform visual acuity tests.	☐	☐	☐	☐	☐
3. Perform extraocular muscle tests.	☐	☐	☐	☐	☐
4. Perform internal (ophthalmoscopic) examination.	☐	☐	☐	☐	☐
Ears					
1. Inspect external ears.	☐	☐	☐	☐	☐
2. Perform internal (otoscopic) examination.	☐	☐	☐	☐	☐
3. Assess hearing acuity.	☐	☐	☐	☐	☐
Thorax and lungs					
1. Inspect shape of thorax and respiratory effort.	☐	☐	☐	☐	☐
2. Percuss the lungs.	☐	☐	☐	☐	☐
3. Auscultate for breath sounds and adventitous sounds.	☐	☐	☐	☐	☐
Breasts					
1. Inspect and palpate breasts (shape, discharge, lesions).	☐	☐	☐	☐	☐
2. Assess stage of sexual development (for girls).	☐	☐	☐	☐	☐
Heart					
1. Inspect and palpate the precordium.	☐	☐	☐	☐	☐
2. Auscultate heart sounds.	☐	☐	☐	☐	☐
Abdomen					
1. Inspect shape.	☐	☐	☐	☐	☐
2. Inspect umbilicus.	☐	☐	☐	☐	☐
3. Auscultate bowel sounds.	☐	☐	☐	☐	☐
4. Palpate softness.	☐	☐	☐	☐	☐
5. Palpate for masses and tenderness.	☐	☐	☐	☐	☐
6. Palpate liver.	☐	☐	☐	☐	☐
7. Palpate spleen.	☐	☐	☐	☐	☐
8. Palpate kidneys.	☐	☐	☐	☐	☐
9. Palpate bladder.	☐	☐	☐	☐	☐
Male Genitalia					
1. Inspect penis and urinary meatus.	☐	☐	☐	☐	☐
2. Inspect and palpate scrotum and testes.	☐	☐	☐	☐	☐

PHYSICAL ASSESSMENT CHECKLIST

Assessment Skill	Findings (Normal or Abnormal) and Notes		Performance (Satisfactory, Needs Improvement, Unsatisfactory)		
	N	A	S	N	U
3. Inspect and palpate inguinal area for hernias.	☐	☐	☐	☐	☐
4. Assess sexual development.	☐	☐	☐	☐	☐
Female Genitalia					
1. Inspect external genitalia.	☐	☐	☐	☐	☐
2. Inspect internal genitalia.	☐	☐	☐	☐	☐
3. Assess sexual development.	☐	☐	☐	☐	☐
Anus and rectum					
1. Inspect anus.	☐	☐	☐	☐	☐
2. Palpate rectum.	☐	☐	☐	☐	☐
Musculoskeletal					
1. Assess feet and legs.	☐	☐	☐	☐	☐
2. Assess for congenital hip dysplasia.	☐	☐	☐	☐	☐
3. Assess spine and posture.	☐	☐	☐	☐	☐
4. Assess gait.	☐	☐	☐	☐	☐
5. Assess joints.	☐	☐	☐	☐	☐
6. Assess muscles.	☐	☐	☐	☐	☐
Neurologic					
1. Perform newborn assessment.	☐	☐	☐	☐	☐
2. Test cerebral function (language, memory, cognition).	☐	☐	☐	☐	☐
3. Test cranial nerve function.	☐	☐	☐	☐	☐
4. Test deep tendon and superficial reflexes.	☐	☐	☐	☐	☐
5. Test balance and coordination.	☐	☐	☐	☐	☐
6. Test sensory function.	☐	☐	☐	☐	☐
7. Test motor function and infantile reflexes.	☐	☐	☐	☐	☐
8. Observe for "soft" signs.	☐	☐	☐	☐	☐
Analysis of data					
1. Formulate nursing diagnoses (wellness, risk, actual).	☐	☐	☐	☐	☐
2. Formulate collaborative problems.	☐	☐	☐	☐	☐
3. Make necessary referrals.	☐	☐	☐	☐	☐

CRITICAL THINKING AND CASE STUDIES

1. On the basis of the following assessment information, work through the steps of analyzing the data. Identify abnormal data and strengths in **subjective and objective findings**, assemble **cue clusters**, draw **inferences**, make possible **nursing diagnoses**, identify **defining characteristics, confirm or rule out** the nursing diagnosis, and **document** your conclusions.

    Use the blank diagnostic analysis charts provided at the end of this book to guide your thinking. You may want to write on the chart or use separate paper.

Propose nursing diagnoses that are specific to the client in the case study. Identify collaborative problems, if any, for this client. Finally, identify data, if any, that point toward a medical problem requiring a referral.

You are the home health nurse assigned to visit 12-year-old Sara Smith, who has mild cerebral palsy and a seizure disorder. Sara has difficulty with gross and fine motor movement and must wear leg braces. However, she is a very intelligent child, who makes up for her disability with her gift for creativity. Recently she has experienced an increase in seizure activity. Her physician has related this to the changes of puberty and has altered her medications. You are making this home visit to see how she is adjusting to her new medications.

During your interview, you find that Sara has just moved to this town. She states that she hates her new house and her new school. She tells you that everyone teases her because of the way she speaks and moves and because of her braces. She also states that she has not told her mother about this because she does not want to upset her. Sara has no siblings. Her mother is a single parent, who works full time and who still expresses some guilt over Sara's "condition," which has existed from birth.

■ Chapter Post-test

MULTIPLE CHOICE QUESTIONS

Choose the one best answer for each of the following multiple-choice questions.

_____ 1. The nurse is assessing a young adolescent female client using Tanner's Sexual Maturity Rating for Breast Development. The nurse determines that the client has enlargement of the breasts and areolae, with no separation of contours. The client is in Tanner Stage

    A. two.

    B. three.

    C. four.

    D. five.

_____ 2. While assessing a young infant's musculoskeletal system, the nurse anticipates that the anterior curve in the lumbar region will be developed by

    A. 6 to 11 months.

    B. 12 to 18 months.

    C. 19 to 24 months.

    D. 25 to 31 months.

_____ 3. A mother brings her 12-year-old son to the clinic for a routine physical. The mother tells the nurse that her son has seemed to be growing taller recently. The nurse should instruct the mother that the peak growth spurt in boys usually occurs by age

    A. 12 years.

    B. 13 years.

C. 14 years.

D. 15 years.

_____ 4. A parent visits the clinic with her 4-year-old child. While communicating with the child, the nurse should

A. touch the child gently but frequently during the interview.

B. stand in front of the child so the child can see the nurse.

C. use standard medical terminology so the child isn't confused.

D. talk to the child in simple terms at the child's eye level.

_____ 5. While communicating with an ill 5-year-old child, one of the most valuable communication techniques that the nurse can use is

A. play.

B. direct communication.

C. indirect communication.

D. closed-ended questions.

_____ 6. A mother visits the clinic with her toddler, who has injured himself in a fall. The nurse caring for the toddler should

A. tell the child it is okay to cry in the clinic.

B. play a game with the child.

C. allow the child to identify the nurse with the parent.

D. use demonstrations when providing health teaching to the child.

_____ 7. The nurse is caring for an 11-year-old child who was hospitalized after an auto accident. While communicating with this child, the nurse should

A. use simple questions.

B. provide simple explanations.

C. use peers as examples.

D. allow the child to engage in the discussions.

_____ 8. The nurse is caring for a hospitalized adolescent with sickle-cell crisis. While communicating with the client, the nurse should

A. give the client control whenever possible.

B. provide simple explanations.

C. use concrete terminology.

D. provide concrete answers to questions.

_____ 9. A mother brings her 4-month-old child to the clinic for subsequent immunizations. The nurse should explain to the mother that at 4 months of age, the recommended immunizations include

A. hepatitis B, DPT, and MMR.

B. oral polio vaccine and MMR.

C. oral polio vaccine, HiB, and DPT.

D. hepatitis B, HiB, and varicella vaccine.

_____ 10. The nurse is assessing a 1-year-old infant who weighed 8 pounds at birth. When the nurse prepares to weigh the infant, the nurse anticipates that this infant should weigh approximately

A. 16 pounds.

B. 20 pounds.

C. 24 pounds.

D. 28 pounds.

_____ 11. A mother visits the clinic for a routine visit with her 5-year-old son. The mother asks the nurse when the child's permanent teeth will erupt. The nurse should explain to the mother that permanent teeth usually begin to erupt by age

A. 5 1/2 years.

A. 6 years.

B. 6 1/2 years.

D. 7 years.

_____ 12. A mother visits the clinic for a routine visit with her 11-year-old daughter. The mother tells the nurse that her daughter has just started puberty. The mother asks the nurse when she can expect the daughter to begin menstruation. The nurse should explain to the mother that menstruation usually begins about

A. 1 year after the onset of puberty.

B. 18 months after the onset of puberty.

C. 24 months after the onset of puberty.

D. 30 months after the onset of puberty.

_____ 13. The nurse is preparing to assess the gross motor development of a 4-year-old child. The nurse should ask the child to

A. hop on one foot.

B. skip a rope.

C. throw a ball.

D. balance on alternate feet with eyes closed.

_____ 14. The nurse is planning to assess the cognitive development of a 3-year-old child. The nurse plans to assess whether or not the child can

A. classify complex objects.

B. quantify objects.

C. sort objects.

D. make simple classifications.

_____ 15. A young mother visits the clinic with her 18-month-old child. The mother asks the nurse when she should begin toilet training with the child. The nurse should explain to the mother that

A. she can begin bowel training as soon as the child appears ready.

B. bladder training usually begins at 18 months of age.

C. nighttime bladder control is usually achieved by 3 years of age.

D. bowel training is usually started when the child is 3 years of age.

_____ 16. A mother visits the clinic with her 2-month-old son for a routine visit. The mother has been bottle-feeding the infant and asks the nurse, "When can I start giving him solid foods?" The nurse should instruct the mother that solid foods can be introduced when the infant is

A. 2 to 4 months old.

B. 4 to 6 months old.

C. 6 to 8 months old.

D. 8 to 10 months old.

_____ 17. The nurse is preparing to assess a 3-month-old child. The mother tells the nurse that the child "tastes salty." The nurse plans to refer the child to a physician for possible

A. cystic fibrosis.

B. kidney disease.

C. gallbladder disease.

D. sweat gland dysfunction.

_____ 18. While assessing a black newborn infant, the nurse observes bluish pigmented areas on the child's buttocks and back. The nurse should

A. document the finding in the client's record.

B. contact a social worker for further assessment of the family.

C. notify the child's pediatrician.

D. assess the child for further evidence of cyanosis.

_____ 19. The nurse is assessing a newborn with the mother present. When the nurse observes an irregularly shaped red patch on the back of the newborn's neck, the nurse should explain to the mother that this is termed

A. port wine stain.

B. hemangioma.

C. cafe au lait spot.

D. storkbite.

_____ 20. While assessing a 4-year-old child, the nurse observes that the child's nails are concave in shape. The nurse should assess the child for a deficiency of

A. magnesium.

B. vitamin C.

C. zinc.

D. iron.

_____ 21. While assessing a newborn infant, the nurse observes yellow-white retention cysts in the newborn's mouth. The nurse should explain to the infant's parents that these spots are usually indicative of

A. Epstein's pearls.

B. thrush.

C. allergic reactions.

D. dehydration.

_____ 22. The nurse is assessing a 4-year-old child with a temperature of 100 degrees F. The nurse observes that the client has Koplik's spots on his buccal mucosa. The nurse should explain to the client's parents that the child is most likely exhibiting signs of

   A. measles.

   B. mumps.

   C. chickenpox.

   D. tonsillitis.

_____ 23. The nurse is preparing to assess a 5-year-old child. To perform the Hirschberg test, the nurse should

   A. ask the child to cover one eye.

   B. shine a light directly into the pupils.

   C. use an ophthalmoscope to check the eyes.

   D. ask the child to name various colors.

_____ 24. The nurse is preparing to inspect a newborn's inner ear with an otoscope. The nurse should pull the pinna

   A. down and back.

   B. up and back.

   C. down and forward.

   D. sideways and forward.

■ Self-Reflection and Evaluation of Learner Objectives

After you have read Chapter 24 and completed the above quizzes and activities, please identify to what degree you have met each of the following chapter learning objectives. For those objectives that you have met partially or not at all, you will want to review chapter content for that learning objective.

Objective	Very much	Somewhat	Not at all
1. Briefly describe how children differ in structure and function from adults, and discuss how these differences affect physical assessment.			
2. Differentiate the interviewing techniques used for parents, infants, toddlers, preschoolers, school-agers, and adolescents.			
3. Explain how play techniques can be used for distraction purposes during assessment.			
4. Explain the components of the pediatric history.			
5. Evaluate the growth and development patterns of infants.			
6. Evaluate the growth and development patterns of toddlers.			
7. Evaluate the growth and development patterns of preschoolers.			

Objective	Very much	Somewhat	Not at all
8. Evaluate the growth and development patterns of school-agers.			
9. Evaluate the growth and development patterns of adolescents.			
10. Describe the components needed in the assessment of the general appearance, and differentiate between norms, variations of normal, and abnormal general appearances.			
11. Demonstrate proper method for assessing vital signs and temperature in infants, children, and adolescents. Discuss the normal ranges for each measurement for infants, children, and adolescents.			
12. Differentiate how heights and weights are assessed in infants and children.			
13. Explain technique used to measure head circumference and why it is measured.			
14. Explain how skin, hair, and nails are assessed, and discuss the possible variations noted in infants, children, and adolescents.			
15. Describe how to assess the head in infants and children, and discuss the norms, variations, and abnormalities that may be noted.			
16. Describe how to assess the face in infants, children, and adolescents, and discuss the norms, variations, and abnormalities that may be noted.			
17. Discuss how to assess the mouth and throat in infants, children, and adolescents, and discuss the norms, variations, and abnormalities that may be noted. Explain proper restraining techniques.			
18. Describe how to assess the nose and sinuses in infants, children, and adolescents, and discuss the norms, variations, and abnormalities that may be noted.			
19. Describe how to assess the eyes and ears in infants, children, and adolescents, and discuss the norms, variations, and abnormalities that may be noted. Differentiate exam techniques between small child and adult (holding pinna for otoscopic exam, visual acuity). Discuss restraining techniques.			

(continues)

(Continued)

Objective	Very much	Somewhat	Not at all
20. Describe how to assess the thorax and lungs in infants, children, and adolescents, and discuss the norms, variations, and abnormalities that may be noted.			
21. Describe how to assess the breasts in infants, children, and adolescents, and discuss the norms, variations, and abnormalities that may be noted. Explain the Tanner stages of female breast development and the method of teaching breast self-examination to adolescents.			
22. Describe how to assess the heart in infants, children, and adolescents, and discuss the norms, variations, and abnormalities that may be noted.			
23. Describe how to assess the abdomen in infants, children, and adolescents, and discuss the norms, variations, and abnormalities that may be noted.			
24. Describe how to assess the male genitalia in infants, children, and adolescents, and discuss the norms, variations, and abnormalities that may be noted. Explain the Tanner stages of male pubic hair and genital development and the method of teaching testicular self-examination to male adolescents.			
25. Describe how to assess the female genitalia in infants, children, and adolescents, and discuss the norms, variations, and abnormalities that may be noted. Explain the Tanner stages of female pubic hair development.			
26. Describe how to assess the anus and rectum in infants, children, and adolescents, and discuss the norms, variations, and abnormalities that may be noted.			
27. Describe how to assess the musculoskeletal system in infants, children, and adolescents, and discuss the norms, variations, and abnormalities that may be noted.			
28. Describe how to assess the neurologic system in infants, children, and adolescents, and discuss the norms, variations, and abnormalities that may be noted. Explain the common infantile reflexes. Explain how the neurologic assessment is integrated into the physical assessment.			

(continues)

Objective	Very much	Somewhat	Not at all
29. Explain how to document and interpret assessment findings.			
30. Discuss various nursing diagnoses and collaborative problems commonly seen with assessment of infants and children.			

For additional information on this book, be sure to visit *http://connection.lww.com.*

Assessment of the Childbearing Woman

CHAPTER OVERVIEW

Women in the childbearing years have unique health care needs, particularly during pregnancy and throughout menopause, when the natural ability to conceive ends. The nursing assessment focuses generally on the various needs and changes specific to women and particularly on the related issues of hormones and hormonal balance.

■ Chapter Pretest

MULTIPLE CHOICE

Choose the one best answer for each of the following multiple-choice questions.

_____ 1. While assessing the abdomen of a pregnant client, the nurse observes striae gravidarum. The nurse should instruct the client that after delivery, the striae gravidarum will

   A. completely disappear.

   B. remain the same.

   C. disappear if a special ointment is used.

   D. fade to a white or silvery color.

_____ 2. While assessing the abdomen of a pregnant woman, the nurse observes a dark line from the client's umbilicus to the mons pubis. The nurse should explain to the client that this is called

   A. linea nigra.

   B. chloasma.

   C. melanin.

   D. epulis.

_____ 3. During pregnancy, a relaxation of the ligaments and joints is caused by the increase in

   A. estrogen.

   B. chorionic gonadotrophin.

   C. lactating hormone.

   D. progesterone.

_____ 4. The nurse is caring for a client who is 24 weeks pregnant. The client tells the nurse that she has been secreting colostrum for the past few days. The nurse should instruct the client that colostrum secretion

A. doesn't normally occur until delivery of the baby.

B. may be indicative of a problem with the breasts.

C. is normal for some women in the second and third trimesters.

D. may be indicative of preterm labor ensuing.

_____ 5. One cardiac change that commonly occurs in a pregnant client is

A. an increase in maternal blood volume by 40 to 50%.

B. a decrease in plasma volume by 20 percent.

C. physiologic hypertension that stabilizes by 24 weeks gestation.

D. a decrease in the heart rate of the client.

_____ 6. As pregnancy progresses, the abdominal muscles may stretch to the point of separation. This condition is termed

A. herniation.

B. McDonald's sign.

C. Goodell's sign.

D. diastasis recti abdominis.

_____ 7. The nurse has instructed a pregnant client about changes that may occur to the client's gastrointestinal system during pregnancy. The nurse determines that the client needs **further** instructions when the client says

A. "As a result of pregnancy, diarrhea may occur more often."

B. "Gastric motility is decreased from the pressure of the fetus."

C. "Constipation may occur because gastric tone is decreased."

D. "Gallstone formation may occur because of prolonged emptying time of the gallbladder."

_____ 8. While interviewing a pregnant client, the nurse determines that the client has pica. The nurse should assess the client's

A. blood sugar.

B. teeth and gums.

C. nutritional status.

D. emotional status.

_____ 9. During pregnancy, the uterus enlarges as a result of hypertrophy of existing myometrial cells and hyperplasia of new cells. This growth is due to

A. estrogen.

B. progesterone.

C. growth hormone.

D. lactating hormone.

_____ 10. The nurse is caring for a pregnant client who is at approximately 20 weeks gestation. The nurse is planning to measure the client's fundal height. At 20 weeks gestation, the nurse should locate the top of the fundus

   A. at the top of the symphysis pubis.

   B. midway between the symphysis pubis and the umbilicus.

   C. at the level of the umbilicus.

   D. above the level of the umbilicus.

■ Learner Activities

After reading Chapter 25, participate in the following learning activities.

CROSSWORD PUZZLE

Complete the following crossword puzzle to become more familiar with the terminology used with assessment of the childbearing woman.

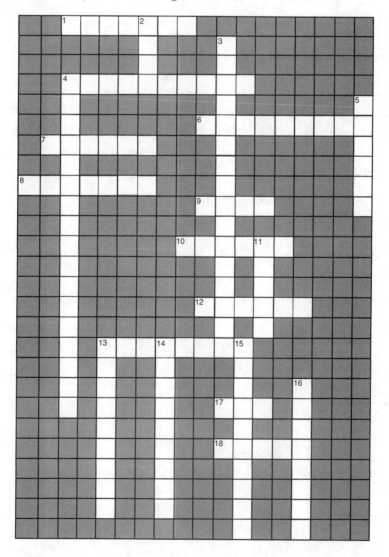

ACROSS

1. Pregnancy in which the ovum is implanted outside the uterine cavity
4. The darker pigmentation appearing on the stomach that extends from the umbilicus to the symphysis pubis
6. The method used to assess uterine contractions
7. Tumor-like lesion that appears on the woman's gums
8. A nonsteroidal hormone that influences the pelvic joints and ligaments to loosen up during pregnancy
9. Fetal heart tones are best heard through the _____ of the fetus.

10. At 30 weeks gestation, the uterus should measure approximately _____ centimeters.
12. The presentation in which the buttocks appear first in the vaginal canal
13. The facial mask of pregnancy
17. In the longitudinal _____ the fetal spine axis is parallel to the mother's spinal axis.
18. True or false: Systolic murmurs are not a normal variant during pregnancy.

DOWN

2. A craving for nonnutritional substances, such as dirt, clay, etc.
3. "Stretch marks" during pregnancy
4. Technique used to determine the presentation, position, and presenting part of the fetus
5. Women may develop physiologic _____ during pregnancy, often because the disproportionate increase in blood volume when compared with red blood cell production.

11. How many trimesters are there in a pregnancy?
13. Fluid secreted from the breasts, especially during the third trimester
14. The _____ conjugate is the smallest opening through which the fetal head must pass.
15. Conflicting feelings and emotions felt by many women during the first trimester
16. Most common type of pelvis found in women

WORKING WITH PEERS IN LEARNING LAB

With a lab partner, role-play nurse and childbearing client. Have the client present with common complaints of pregnancy. Have the nurse reassure the client, explain in layperson's terms the reasons for these symptoms, and offer recommendations for relief. (Also have the nurse refer any problems that are not normal to an appropriate health care provider, such as a midwife or a physician.)

INTERVIEWING AND RECORDING ASSESSMENT FINDINGS

Use the following Nursing History Checklist as your guide for interviewing and recording the findings in an assessment of the childbearing woman.

NURSING HISTORY CHECKLIST

Questions	Satisfactory data	Needs additional data	Data missing
Current Symptoms			
1. Weight changes?			
2. Upper respiratory symptoms?			
3. Stomach or bowel problems?			
4. Urinary tract symptoms?			
5. Vaginal discharge, bleeding, or leaking fluid?			
6. Psychologic problems?			
7. Breast changes?			

(continues)

NURSING HISTORY CHECKLIST *(Continued)*

Questions	Satisfactory data	Needs additional data	Data missing

Past History

1. Past pregnancy history (include all previous deliveries and miscarriages)?
2. Neonatal problems at delivery or within the first 2 weeks of life?
3. Complicated pregnancies requiring termination, molar pregnancy, ectopic pregnancy, etc.?
4. LMP and duration, bleeding since that time?
5. Type of birth control used, if any?
6. Infertility problems?
7. Reproductive surgeries, abnormal Pap smears, etc.?
8. History of sexually transmitted diseases, treatment, vaginal infections, etc.?
9. Blood type?
10. Medical history?
11. Hospitalizations?
12. Surgeries?

Family History

1. History of birth defects in the family?
2. Ethnic background?
3. Heart disease, lung disease, diabetes, asthma, cancer, birth defects, blood disorders, mental retardation, sickle-cell disease?

Lifestyle and Health Practices

1. Age at delivery?
2. Current medications?
3. Alcohol/cigarette use?
4. Street drug use?
5. Family members that consider social habits to be a problem?
6. Diet evaluation?
7. Weight/baseline?
8. Exercise routine?
9. Client's occupation/highest degree?
10. Work routine?
11. Chemical/radiation exposure?
12. Risk for toxoplasmosis?
13. Partner profile?
14. Social support systems?
15. Siblings?

PERFORMING PHYSICAL ASSESSMENT

Use the following Physical Assessment Checklist as your guide to performing an assessment examination of the childbearing woman.

PHYSICAL ASSESSMENT CHECKLIST

Assessment Skill	Findings (Normal or Abnormal) and Notes		Performance (Satisfactory, Needs Improvement, Unsatisfactory)		
	N	A	S	N	U
1. Gather equipment (ophthalmoscope, otoscope, stethoscope, speculum, sphygmomanometer, light, tape measure, fetal Doppler, gloves, lubricant, slides).	☐	☐	☐	☐	☐
2. Explain procedure to client.	☐	☐	☐	☐	☐
3. Ask client to gown.	☐	☐	☐	☐	☐
4. Assess vital signs.	☐	☐	☐	☐	☐
5. Measure weight/height.	☐	☐	☐	☐	☐
6. Observe behavior.	☐	☐	☐	☐	☐
7. Inspect skin.	☐	☐	☐	☐	☐
8. Inspect hair/nails.	☐	☐	☐	☐	☐
9. Inspect neck.	☐	☐	☐	☐	☐
10. Inspect mouth/nose/throat.	☐	☐	☐	☐	☐
11. Inspect, palpate, percuss, and auscultate chest.	☐	☐	☐	☐	☐
12. Inspect and palpate breasts.	☐	☐	☐	☐	☐
13. Auscultate heart.	☐	☐	☐	☐	☐
14. Inspect and palpate abdomen.	☐	☐	☐	☐	☐
15. Measure fundal height.	☐	☐	☐	☐	☐
16. Assess fetal position.	☐	☐	☐	☐	☐
17. Auscultate fetal heart tones.	☐	☐	☐	☐	☐
18. Inspect external genitalia.	☐	☐	☐	☐	☐
19. Palpate Bartholin's and Skene's glands.	☐	☐	☐	☐	☐
20. Inspect vaginal opening.	☐	☐	☐	☐	☐
21. Perform speculum examination.	☐	☐	☐	☐	☐
22. Obtain specimens.	☐	☐	☐	☐	☐
23. Perform pelvic examination.	☐	☐	☐	☐	☐
24. Inspect anus/rectum.	☐	☐	☐	☐	☐
25. Auscultate blood pressure.	☐	☐	☐	☐	☐
26. Inspect face and extremities.	☐	☐	☐	☐	☐
27. Percuss deep tendon reflexes.	☐	☐	☐	☐	☐
28. Determine pelvic adequacy.	☐	☐	☐	☐	☐
29. Determine height/inclination of symphysis pubis.	☐	☐	☐	☐	☐
30. Palpate lateral walls of pelvis.	☐	☐	☐	☐	☐
31. Palpate ischial spines.	☐	☐	☐	☐	☐
32. Palpate sacrum/coccyx.	☐	☐	☐	☐	☐

(continues)

PHYSICAL ASSESSMENT CHECKLIST

Assessment Skill	Findings (Normal or Abnormal) and Notes		Performance (Satisfactory, Needs Improvement, Unsatisfactory)		
	N	A	S	N	U
33. Measure diagonal conjugate.	☐	☐	☐	☐	☐
34. Calculate obstetric conjugate.	☐	☐	☐	☐	☐
35. Measure transverse diameter of the pelvic outlet.	☐	☐	☐	☐	☐
36. Assess for complaints of common neurologic discomforts during pregnancy.	☐	☐	☐	☐	☐
37. Formulate nursing diagnoses (wellness, risk, actual).	☐	☐	☐	☐	☐
38. Formulate collaborative problems.	☐	☐	☐	☐	☐
39. Make necessary referrals.	☐	☐	☐	☐	☐

CRITICAL THINKING AND CASE STUDIES

1. On the basis of the following assessment information, work through the steps of analyzing the data. Identify abnormal data and strengths in **subjective and objective findings**, assemble **cue clusters**, draw **inferences**, make possible **nursing diagnoses**, identify **defining characteristics**, **confirm or rule out** the nursing diagnosis, and **document** your conclusions.

   Use the blank diagnostic analysis charts provided at the end of this book to guide your thinking. You may want to write on the chart or use separate paper. Propose nursing diagnoses that are specific to the client in the case study. Identify collaborative problems, if any, for this client. Finally, identify data, if any, that point toward a medical problem requiring a referral.

   Kaitlin presents to your office today, thinking that she may be pregnant. Kaitlin is a 20-year-old primigravida who remembers her last menstrual period (LMP) as having been March 13, 2002, which would make her at approximately 20 weeks gestation. She states that she did have some irregular spotting in April for approximately 2 days.

   Kaitlin's medical and surgical history is unremarkable. Her family history is also noncontributory. Her social history is negative for alcohol and drugs. She is single and lives at home with her parents while attending college. The father of the baby is involved but is unsure about his feelings regarding the pregnancy. This pregnancy was not planned, and he wants to finish college and develop his career. Marriage plans are not in the father's schedule at this time.

■ Chapter Post-test

MULTIPLE CHOICE QUESTIONS

Choose the one best answer for each of the following multiple-choice questions.

_____ 1. A pregnant client who is at approximately 36 weeks gestation tells the nurse that she experiences dizziness while in bed. The nurse should instruct the client to avoid which position?

A. side-lying

B. left lateral

C. prone

D. supine

_____ 2. A client who is of normal weight just learned that she is 10 weeks pregnant. The client asks the nurse about weight gain during pregnancy. The nurse should instruct the client that the recommended weight gain is

A. 15 to 20 pounds.

B. 20 to 25 pounds.

C. 25 to 35 pounds.

D. 35 to 45 pounds.

_____ 3. A pregnant client at 12 weeks gestation visits the clinic and tells the nurse that she has been vomiting severely for the past 5 days. The nurse should refer the client to a physician for possible

A. hyperemesis gravidarum.

B. viral infection.

C. fetal anomalies.

D. peptic ulcer.

_____ 4. A pregnant client visits the clinic for the first time. She tells the nurse that she has had two spontaneous miscarriages before this pregnancy. The nurse should refer the client to a physician for possible

A. incompetent cervix.

B. substance abuse.

C. Rh incompatibility.

D. hyperthyroidism.

_____ 5. A pregnant client visits the clinic for the first time. The client tells the nurse that this is her first pregnancy and that she and her husband are Ashkenazi Jews and immigrated to the United States from Israel. The nurse should encourage the client to be tested for

A. sickle-cell anemia.

B. cystic fibrosis.

C. cerebral palsy.

D. Tay-Sachs disease.

_____ 6. A pregnant client near term is admitted to the hospital with scant vaginal bleeding and mild contractions. The client tells the nurse that she uses cocaine occasionally. The nurse should assess the client for signs and symptoms of

   A. oligohydramnios.

   B. polyhydramnios.

   C. placenta previa.

   D. abruptio placenta.

_____ 7. A pregnant client visits the clinic for the first time. The nurse should explain to the client that she will have initial routine blood tests, which include testing for

   A. alpha-fetoprotein levels.

   B. chromosomal anomalies.

   C. cystic fibrosis.

   D. Rh status.

_____ 8. A pregnant client visits the clinic at 36 weeks gestation. The nurse weighs the client and determines that the client has gained 5 pounds in 1 week. The nurse should assess the client's

   A. dietary patterns.

   B. edema of the lower extremities.

   C. urinary patterns.

   D. blood pressure.

_____ 9. The nurse is planning to perform Leopold's maneuvers on a pregnant client. To perform the first maneuver, the nurse should place his or her hands on the

   A. upper quadrant of the maternal abdomen.

   B. lateral sides of the maternal abdomen.

   C. presenting part.

   D. top of the symphysis pubis.

_____ 10. While caring for a pregnant client at 8 weeks gestation, the client asks the nurse, "When can you hear the baby's heartbeat?" The nurse should instruct the client that when a Doppler device is used, the earliest time when the fetal heart rate can be heard is the gestational age of

   A. 10 weeks.

   B. 14 weeks.

   C. 18 weeks.

   D. 22 weeks.

_____ 11. While assessing a pregnant client, the nurse detects fetal heart rate decelerations that occur after a contraction. The nurse should notify the client's physician because this may be indicative of

   A. fetal demise.

   B. cardiac disease.

   C. head compression.

   D. poor placental perfusion.

_____ 12. The nurse is preparing to assess the fetal heart rate of a pregnant client near term. When the nurse hears the fetal heart rate above the maternal umbilicus, the fetus is most likely in which position?

A. transverse

B. breech

C. vertex

D. face

_____ 13. A pregnant client visits the clinic and complains of a thick, purulent vaginal discharge. The nurse should obtain a specimen of the vaginal discharge because this type of discharge is usually indicative of

A. gonorrhea.

B. bacterial vaginosis.

C. _Candida albicans_ infection.

D. chlamydial infection .

_____ 14. While assessing a pregnant client at 36 weeks gestation, the nurse observes that the client's face is edematous and she has 3+ reflexes with mild clonus. The nurse should refer the client to a physician for possible

A. hydatidiform mole.

B. multiple gestation.

C. pregnancy-induced hypertension.

D. hyperthyroidism.

_____ 15. The nurse is caring for a pregnant client at 14 weeks gestation and determines that the measurement between the client's ischial tuberosities is 10.5 centimeters. The nurse should

A. instruct the client that a vaginal delivery is likely.

B. refer the client to a physician for small pelvic size.

C. measure the pubic arch to validate the measurement.

D. estimate the size of the fetus.

■ Self-Reflection and Evaluation of Learner Objectives

After you have read Chapter 25 and completed the above quizzes and activities, please identify to what degree you have met each of the following chapter learning objectives. For those objectives that you have met partially or not at all, you will want to review chapter content for that learning objective.

Objective	Very much	Somewhat	Not at all
1. Explain the dynamic cardiovascular changes that occur during pregnancy.			
2. Describe the skin changes that occur during pregnancy.			
3. Measure the progressional growth of the uterus during pregnancy.			
4. Discuss common concerns and complaints experienced by the pregnant client.			
5. Obtain an accurate nursing history by conducting a prenatal interview.			
6. Demonstrate how to correctly perform Leopold's maneuvers.			

For additional information on this book, be sure to visit *http://connection.lww.com.*

Assessment of the Frail Elderly Adult

CHAPTER OVERVIEW

What distinguishes a frail elderly adult from an elderly adult is his or her delicate balance of health and independence, which can easily be compromised by a disease or a minor accident.

■ Chapter Pretest

MULTIPLE CHOICE

Choose the one best answer for each of the following multiple-choice questions.

_____ 1. The physical declines of aging often first become noticeable when
   A. approximately 50% of function is lost.
   B. the person is at least 75 years old.
   C. acute or chronic illness places excessive demands on the body.
   D. cognitive declines become significant.

_____ 2. A benign skin lesion commonly seen in the aged is
   A. squamous cell carcinoma.
   B. shingles.
   C. actinic keratosis.
   D. lentigo.

_____ 3. Diminished vibratory sensations and slowed motor responses in advanced age result in
   A. stiffness and rigidity.
   B. paresthesia.
   C. postural instability.
   D. tremors.

_____ 4. A sign of infection in the elder that is more common than fever is
   A. pain.
   B. confusion.
   C. diarrhea.
   D. cough.

_____ 5. By age 90, renal blood flow has usually decreased by approximately
   A. 5%.
   B. 10%.
   C. 25%.
   D. 50%.

_____ 6. A neurologic change associated with normal aging is
   A. loss of long-term memory.
   B. a decrease in reaction time.
   C. swaying or shuffling gait.
   D. a significant decline in judgment and cognition.

MATCHING

Match the terms in the left column with the correct descriptions in the right column.

Term	Description
_____ 1. Calcification, stiffening, and dilation of the aortic valve	A. Rise in systolic blood pressure
_____ 2. Decreased ventricular compliance	B. Soft systolic murmur at base of heart
_____ 3. Loss of elasticity in aorta and arteries	C. S_4
_____ 4. Decreased baroreceptor sensitivity	D. Orthostatic hypotension

■ Learner Activities

After reading Chapter 26, participate in the following learning activities.

WORKING WITH PEERS IN LEARNING LAB

1. Practice the timed Get Up and Go test on your lab partner. Then do the test again with your lab partner, using crutches to walk. Do it one more time with your partner's arm in a sling. How do these disabilities affect gait stability and timing?

2. Identify and discuss with your lab partner two risk factors for each problem included in the acronym SPICES.

3. Find a frail elder 80 years or older who is not completely independent in some aspect of everyday life. Assess the degree to which he or she is dependent in activities of daily living (ADLs) and instrumental activities of daily living (IADLs). Also address this person's physical and social environment for barriers and for resources related to independent function.

4. Visit a retail supplier of rehabilitative aids or home medical equipment. Locate items that assist persons with various degrees of immobility. Itemize at least 10 of them from least to most expensive.

5. Visit an intensive care unit. Identify as many factors as you can in the physical environment or the nursing practices that may contribute to delirium in a frail elder.

6. Review the medication profile of five hospitalized elders over the age of 80. Identify all the medications they are taking that have anticholinergic side effects. Describe the assessment parameters that are indicated.

INTERVIEWING AND RECORDING ASSESSMENT FINDINGS

Use the following Functional Status Checklist as your guide to adapting the nursing health history and physical examination for the frail elder client. Record your findings.

FUNCTIONAL STATUS CHECKLIST

Function	Findings

Activities of Daily Living (ADLs)

1. Bathing
2. Eating
3. Dressing
4. Toileting
5. Transferring
6. Walking

Instrumental Activities of Daily Living (IADLs)

1. Shopping
2. Meal preparation
3. Housekeeping
4. Transportation
5. Money management
6. Ability to use the telephone
7. Medication management

Geriatric Syndromes

1. Skin impairment
2. Poor nutrition
3. Incontinence
4. Cognitive impairment
5. Evidence of falls or functional decline
6. Sleep disturbances

Special Tests Indicated by History or Physical Examination

1. Assessment of swallowing
2. Voice-whisper examination
3. Get Up and Go test
4. 24-hour food and fluid diary
5. Mini-Nutritional Assessment
6. Mini-Mental State Exam
7. Geriatric depression scale
8. Assessment of urinary continence

CRITICAL THINKING AND CASE STUDIES

1. Explain the various ways in which falls or a history of falls should be assessed in the frail elder.

2. Identify an acute pathologic condition that may manifest as a decline in functional ability. Explain how you might identify the condition, and describe the appropriate actions to take once it has been identified.

3. Compare and contrast the steps of a musculoskeletal and neurologic examination of a young adult with those for an adult over the age of 85. Pay close attention to the significance of those steps that assess functional status.

4. You are a nurse in the emergency room. An 88-year-old woman is brought in by her daughter-in-law. Upon initial examination, you notice that this thin, frail, elderly woman has bruises on her back, buttocks, and upper chest. She follows your actions with her eyes, but mainly groans or cries out, "Oh take it away. . . take it away." When you try to find out why she has been brought to the E.R. today, her daughter-in-law tells you that the client fell in the bathtub and she's worried that she may have broken a bone.

   How would you adjust the interview to adapt to the needs of this elderly woman? Describe key features of the musculoskeletal and neurologic exams that need to be undertaken. What aspects of a functional and psychosocial assessment should you perform?

■ Chapter Post-test

MULTIPLE CHOICE

Choose the one best answer for each of the following multiple-choice questions.

_____ 1. A risk factor for sinusitis in the frail elderly is
   A. a nasogastric feeding tube
   B. an accumulation of ear wax
   C. decreased ability to detect odors
   D. conductive hearing loss

_____ 2. Common signs or symptoms of disease in the oldest-old include all of the below *except*
   A. weakness.
   B. confusion.
   C. falls.
   D. fever.

_____ 3. Any new onset of incontinence in the frail elder should be investigated for
   A. prostatitis.
   B. stroke.
   C. fecal impaction.
   D. urinary tract infection.

_____ 4. An objective assessment that is frequently indicated when the subjective assessment reveals a history of falling is

    A. a 24-hour food diary.

    B. a Get Up and Go test.

    C. a tonometry exam.

    D. palpation of the joints for crepitus.

_____ 5. A gastrointestinal problem that often requires emergency treatment in the frail elder is

    A. lactose intolerance.

    B. hiatal hernia.

    C. diverticulitis.

    D. Crohn's disease.

_____ 6. To compensate for a stooped posture and less flexible knee, hip, and shoulder joints, the elderly person often walks

    A. with a waddling type of gait.

    B. with one leg slightly dragging behind the other.

    C. with the feet farther apart and the knees slightly bent.

    D. with a slight swaying side-to-side motion.

_____ 7. A common sign or symptom of depression in the elderly is

    A. rambling or incoherent speech.

    B. illusion or hallucinations.

    C. insomnia.

    D. cognitive impairment or pseudodementia.

_____ 8. A key area to assess in older adults with chronic respiratory or cardiac problems and some constant degree of dyspnea is

    A. nutritional deficiency.

    B. dysphagia.

    C. the degree to which dyspnea affects daily function.

    D. a possible history of immunosuppression.

_____ 9. A characteristic sign of delirium is

    A. a significant decline in memory.

    B. a chronic low mood.

    C. a rapid decline in level of alertness.

    D. disorientation to self.

_____ 10. All of the following are accurate signs of dehydration in the frail elder _except_

    A. a furrowed tongue.

    B. tenting of the skin when pinched.

    C. dry, warm skin.

    D. sunken eyes.

_____ 11. Signs of arterial insufficiency in the very old include all of the
        following *except*

   A. paleness of the leg when elevated.

   B. dusky or mottled appearance of the leg in a dependent position.

   C. hair loss on the skin.

   D. cool, thin, shiny skin.

MATCHING

*In Part 1, match the sign or symptom with the corresponding eye disorder (only one
response per question). In Part 2, match the medication with the adverse side effect
that it may cause (possibly more than one answer per question; some responses may
not be used at all).*

PART 1. EYE SYMPTOMS AND DISORDERS

_____ 1. Noticeable loss of vision and distortion
          of familiar objects, and occasional floaters

_____ 2. Floaters associated with flashes of light

_____ 3. Blurriness of words in center of the page

_____ 4. Significant decrease in central vision

PART 2. MEDICATIONS AND ADVERSE EFFECTS

_____ 5. Whitish or yellow-tinged patches in mouth

_____ 6. Orthostatic hypotension

_____ 7. Erectile dysfunction

_____ 8. GI bleeding

_____ 9. Constipation

A. macular degeneration

B. retinal detachment

C. cataract

D. diabetic retinopathy

E. oral corticosteroid

F. steroidal inhalant

G. antidepressants

H. anticoagulants

I. anticholinergics

J. antihypertensives

■ Self-Reflection and Evaluation
of Learner Objectives

After you have read Chapter 26 and completed the above quizzes and activities,
please identify to what degree you have met each of the following chapter learning
objectives. For those objectives that you have met partially or not at all, you will
want to review chapter content for that learning objective.

Objective	Very much	Somewhat	Not at all
1. Describe the common structural changes brought on by aging in the various body systems.			
2. Recognize the unique presentation of disease and illness in the very old (often referred to as the geriatric syndromes).			
3. Effectively interview the frail elderly client by modifying interview techniques used for the adult client.			

Objective	Very much	Somewhat	Not at all
4. Effectively examine the frail elderly client by modifying the physical examination techniques used for the adult client.			
5. Describe assessment abnormalities in the frail elderly client that may be the result of adverse drug effects.			
6. Explain how to incorporate assessment of functional status when collecting subjective and objective data on the frail elderly client to accurately evaluate findings.			

For additional information on this book, be sure to visit *http://connection.lww.com.*

Assessment of the Family

CHAPTER OVERVIEW

In assessing the family, many nurses focus on the individual as client and the family as context for the client's health and care. This requires assessing family strengths and problem areas as they affect the family support system. If the whole family is viewed as the client, then nursing assessment is directed toward the family unit as a dynamic system.

■ Chapter Pretest

MULTIPLE CHOICE

Choose the one best answer for each of the following multiple-choice questions.

_____ 1. A broad definition of the family includes two or more persons who
   A. are related by blood.
   B. live in the same household.
   C. are married.
   D. have mutual decision making.

_____ 2. The internal structure of a family includes
   A. the gender of the members.
   B. ethnic identity.
   C. religious practices.
   D. social class.

_____ 3. An example of a subsystem of a family is
   A. father—-renter.
   B. mother—-chairperson.
   C. father—-leader.
   D. mother—-son.

_____ 4. According to the theory by Minuchin, disengaged families have boundaries that are
   A. open.
   B. diffuse.
   C. permeable.
   D. rigid.

_____ 5. In the most functional families, parents have power that
   A. rests with the father.
   B. rests with the mother.
   C. is shared by both parents.
   D. is shared by all of the family members.

Matching

Match the terms in the left column with the correct descriptions in the right column.

Term	Description
_____ 1. Ecomap	A. Feedback system of reciprocal communication between people
_____ 2. Self-differentiation	B. Similarity of illness or behaviors that run through the family from one generation to the next
_____ 3. Circular communication	C. Diagram of the family's contact with larger systems
_____ 4. Gender role	D. Behaviors expected of family members based on their sex and family beliefs about masculinity and femininity
_____ 5. Multigenerational patterns	E. Young adult's shift toward separation from the family of origin

■ Learner Activities

After reading Chapter 27, participate in the following learning activities.

WORKING WITH PEERS IN LEARNING LAB

1. Have a group of lab partners make lists of words that each associates with family. Discuss the patterns and definitions of family revealed by the words.

2. Determine your family's life-cycle stage based on the stage of the American family in Chapter 27.

3. Make a genogram of your family over three or four generations. Add causes and dates of illness or death for each family member. Note any repeating patterns.

INTERVIEWING AND RECORDING ASSESSMENT FINDINGS

Use the following Nursing History Checklist as your guide to interviewing a peer and recording your findings in a family assessment.

NURSING HISTORY CHECKLIST

Questions	Normal findings	Abnormal findings	Data missing
Internal Family Structure			
1. Construct genogram of family composition.			
2. Family type and who is considered to be family.			
3. Recent movement in or out.			
4. Gender role.			
5. Rank order.			
6. Family subsystems.			
7. Family boundaries (permeable, rigid, or diffuse).			
8. Family power structure.			
External Family Structure			
1. Construct an ecomap.			
2. Extended family.			
3. External systems.			
4. Context.			
Family Development			
1. Life cycle stages and tasks.			
Instrumental Function			
1. Ability to carry out activities of daily living.			
Affective and Socialization Function			
1. Support and nurturance of family members.			
2. Parenting practices for socialization of children.			
3. Subgroups for triangles and boundaries (permeable, rigid, diffuse boundaries; level of self-differentiation of family members).			
Expressive Function			
1. Construct a family attachment diagram.			
2. Emotional communication.			
3. Verbal communication.			
4. Nonverbal communication.			
5. Circular communication.			
Health Care Function			
1. Family's health care function (beliefs and practices).			

NURSING HISTORY CHECKLIST

Questions	Normal findings	Abnormal findings	Data missing
Multigenerational Patterns			
1. Data for multigenerational patterns of positive and negative behaviors.			
Analysis of Data			
1. Formulate nursing diagnoses (wellness, risk, actual).			
2. Formulate collaborative problems (if present).			
3. Make necessary referrals.			

CRITICAL THINKING AND CASE STUDIES

1. On the basis of the following assessment information, work through the steps of analyzing the data. Identify abnormal data and strengths in **subjective and objective** findings, assemble **cue clusters, draw inferences**, make possible **nursing diagnoses**, identify **defining characteristics, confirm or rule out** the nursing diagnosis, and **document** your conclusions.

   Use the blank diagnostic analysis charts provided at the end of this book to guide your thinking. You may want to write on the chart or use separate paper. Propose nursing diagnoses that are specific to the client in the case study. Identify collaborative problems, if any, for this client. Finally, identify data, if any, that point toward a medical problem requiring a referral.

   The Harrison family has come to the clinic for a renewal of prescriptions. Mary Harrison begins to talk to the nurse about the increasing stress that she is under because of her parents' illnesses. In the course of the conversation, the nurse asks whether Mary believes that she and the family need help with deciding how to handle the many problems associated with caring for her mother with Alzheimer's disease and her father with congestive heart failure. The Harrison family decides to arrange to meet with the nurse to discuss these problems.

   The Harrison family is composed of a couple (Mary and Richard), Mary's mother and father (Nan and Ned), and two grown children (Maria and Stan), who live and work in other cities. Mary is a 52-year-old schoolteacher who has had to take a leave of absence to care for her mother, Nan. Nan is 78 years old and has advancing Alzheimer's disease. Richard, 53 years old, works in construction and on occasion is out of work. Ned is 80 years old and has congestive heart failure, which makes it difficult for him to care for his wife. Nan and Ned moved in with Mary and Richard when Maria and Stan moved away 2 years ago. Financial pressures are increasing because of Mary's 3-month leave of absence and Richard's variable annual income. Nan and Ned have no income other than Ned's social security.

   Mary describes herself as less and less able to keep up with the house, the meals, and her mother's personal care needs. Richard says that Mary is becoming very grouchy and unpleasant and that she rarely wants to have sex. Mary accuses Richard of not doing anything to help her around the house. Richard says that housework and caring for people is women's work. No one in the family wants to put Nan in a nursing home.

■ Chapter Post-test

MULTIPLE CHOICE QUESTIONS

Choose the one best answer for each of the following multiple-choice questions.

_____ 1. The nurse is preparing to draw a genogram of a client's family. The symbol for male members of the family is a
   A. triangle.
   B. circle.
   C. oval.
   D. square.

_____ 2. One element of the context of a family's structure is
   A. ethnicity.
   B. extended family members.
   C. gender.
   D. power.

_____ 3. The ability of a family to carry out activities of daily living is a family function termed
   A. employment.
   B. exchanging.
   C. differentiation.
   D. instrumental.

_____ 4. According to Bowen's family theory, differentiation of self is assessed by
   A. determining the number of members in the family.
   B. looking at the communication patterns of the family.
   C. documenting the roles of each family member.
   D. determining the boundaries of the subsystems in the family structure.

_____ 5. Families with moderately differentiated members will exhibit
   A. rigid patterns of interactions.
   B. difficulties in delaying gratification.
   C. difficulties in maintaining intimate personal relations.
   D. family roles that are based on skills and interests.

_____ 6. Cybernetics, as applied to families, combines communication with
   A. Minuchin's theory.
   B. general systems theory.
   C. Friedman's theory.
   D. Bowen's theory.

_____ 7. One example of a complementary birth order of spouses is
   A. youngest son marries youngest daughter.
   B. middle son marries middle daughter.

    C. oldest son marries youngest daughter.

    D. oldest son marries oldest daughter.

_____ 8. In the assessment of the family's home environment, an important characteristic for the nurse to assess is the

    A. neighborhood's safety.

    B. school system.

    C. public transportation.

    D. availability of churches.

_____ 9. While assessing a family, the nurse determines that the family's parental practices are based on control, coercion, and punishment. These parenting practices discourage

    A. self-fulfillment.

    B. self-differentiation.

    C. circular communication.

    D. socialization.

_____ 10. The nurse visits a family at home after the 16-year-old only son was injured severely in an automobile accident. The client is in a wheelchair and requires 24-hour care. The client's mother is the sole caregiver, and she tells the nurse that she is saddened because "my son was such a wonderful basketball player." A priority family nursing diagnosis is

    A. depression related to youthful family member's health status.

    B. ineffective community coping related to mother being sole caregiver.

    C. immobility related to severe injuries from automobile accident.

    D. risk for dysfunctional grieving related to loss of health status of youthful family member.

MATCHING

Match the terms in the left column with the correct descriptions in the right column.

Term	Description
_____ 1. Genogram	A. Messages sent through body position, eye contact, touch, gestures, tone of voice, crying, or stammering, etc.
_____ 2. Nuclear family	B. The position of the children within a family based on age and gender
_____ 3. Rank order	
_____ 4. Emotional communication	C. The range and types of feelings that are openly expressed or acceptable to be communicated within a family
_____ 5. Nonverbal communication	
	D. A diagram of the family tree showing genetics, generational information, and relationships of family members
	E. Usually considered to include father, mother, and children

■ Self-Reflection and Evaluation of Learner Objectives

After you have read Chapter 27 and completed the above quizzes and activities, please identify to what degree you have met each of the following chapter learning objectives. For those objectives that you have met partially or not at all, you will want to review chapter content for that learning objective.

Objective	Very much	Somewhat	Not at all
1. Define *family*.			
2. List the three essential components of a family assessment (structure, development, and function) and the major elements of each component.			
3. Determine a family's life cycle stage and the related tasks.			
4. Construct a genogram for a three-generational family.			
5. Construct a family attachment diagram.			
6. Construct a family ecomap.			
7. Discuss theoretic concepts of family function, including systems theory, Bowen's family system theory, and communication theory.			
8. Use Bowen's theory to determine the level of self-differentiation of a family and its members and to detect triangles within a family.			
9. Describe the importance of communication to family function.			
10. Discuss various nursing diagnoses and collaborative problems commonly seen with assessment of the family.			

For additional information on this book, be sure to visit *http://connection.lww.com*.

Assessment of the Community

CHAPTER OVERVIEW

Community may be defined and classified in various ways depending on one's perspective. A nursing assessment of a community, however, aims to determine the health-related concerns of its members, regardless of the type of the community.

■ Chapter Pretest

MULTIPLE CHOICE

Choose the one best answer for each of the following multiple-choice questions.

_____ 1. In 1993, the number one cause of childhood mortality in the United States for children between the ages of 5 and 14 years was

    A. malignant neoplasms.

    B. congenital anomalies.

    C. motor vehicle accidents.

    D. burns.

_____ 2. In 1994, the number one cause of mortality in the United States for people between the ages of 45 and 64 was

    A. stroke.

    B. heart disease.

    C. accidents.

    D. cancer.

_____ 3. In 1994, the number one cause of mortality in the United States for people 65 and older was

    A. heart disease.

    B. cancer.

    C. stroke.

    D. accidents.

_____ 4. Since 1970, the number of divorces in the United States has

    A. declined.

    B. doubled.

    C. tripled.

    D. quadrupled.

_____ 5. In the United States, single parents are at a greater risk for health problems, especially those related to

A. finances.

B. housing.

C. role overload.

D. basic needs.

_____ 6. In the United States, the growing number of homeless individuals and families is related to the community's

A. disregard for these individuals.

B. lack of resources for assistance.

C. high unemployment rates.

D. lack of affordable housing.

_____ 7. Many communities, especially those in rural areas, cannot provide needed health care services, particularly those related to

A. cardiac care.

B. orthopedic care.

C. dental care.

D. obstetric care.

_____ 8. The fastest-growing components of the health care system in the United States are

A. wellness clinics.

B. pediatric clinics.

C. long-term institutional care facilities.

D. home health care agencies.

_____ 9. In rural areas of the United States, one major problem that makes many social service programs inaccessible is

A. a lack of community awareness.

B. reliance on federal support monies.

C. a lack of transportation.

D. a limited number of welfare programs.

_____ 10. One major condition that is associated with higher morbidity and mortality rates in a community is

A. the educational level.

B. the number of health care facilities.

C. the religious beliefs of the population.

D. poverty.

CROSSWORD PUZZLE

Complete the following crossword puzzle to become more familiar with the terminology used with assessment of the community.

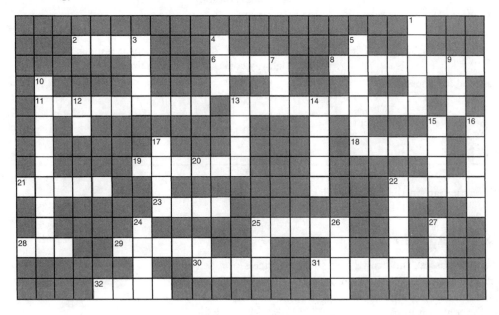

ACROSS

2. Community recreation programs usually provide for both individual and _____ sports.

6. A weather-related condition often associated with accidents and other health problems

8. Food _____ are often provided by local religious organizations.

11. Another term for "disease" data

13. A type of anemia prevalent in African Americans

18. A natural boundary often used to separate geographic regions

19. U.S. department where demographic information may be obtained

21. U.S. department involved in data collection related to unemployment information

22. A title that may be given to the chief elected official of a city or town

23. Program available through some local police departments, designed to help combat drug use among adolescents

25. Birth and death records are examples of _____ statistics.

28. Abbreviation for degree awarded to an individual who did not complete high school but later returns to classes to receive a diploma

29. Disposal of hazardous _____ is a serious environmental concern for many communities.

30. A voluntary agency that provides social programs and activities for children and adults (abbreviation)

31. An economical means of transportation available in many large urban areas is rapid _____.

32. A body of water that often provides a site for recreation in many communities

DOWN

1. Access to health care is a concern to those in remote _____ areas.

3. A community group organized to combat driving under the influence of alcohol (acronym)

4. Abbreviation for Social Security Administration

5. Leading cause of death in U.S. adults aged 45-54

7. Federal program designed to provide nutritional supplements and education for women and children (acronym)

9. Federal agency responsible for environmental concerns (abbreviation)

10. A component of emergency care, which may not be available in some rural areas

12. An abbreviation associated with train travel

13. Second leading cause of infant mortality in the United States in 1991 (acronym)

14. A tick-borne illness associated with certain geographic regions of the United States

15. A voluntary agency found in many areas is the Salvation _____.

16. A means of communication in many small towns is a community bulletin _____.

17. Type of poisoning often associated with ingestion of paint from older homes

20. A method of collecting information from large numbers of people

22. A program that provides food for homebound individuals is _____ on Wheels.

24. An area in a community where many recreational activities are held

25. An example of a nonprofit agency that provides home care (abbreviation)

26. Stories about the history of a community may be referred to as local _____.

27. Abbreviation for state department responsible for highway construction and maintenance

■ Learner Activities

After reading Chapter 28, participate in the following learning activities.

WORKING WITH PEERS IN LEARNING LAB

1. With a group of lab partners, assess the health and social service s of a selected part of your community. Include items 1 through 5 on the Community Assessment Checklist below. Discuss your findings regarding whether the resources are adequate for that community.

2. With a group of lab partners, have each group member take a specific age group and list the forms of recreation that might be of interest to that age group and how form of recreation might contribute to health.

3. Go to an inner-city health clinic or a rural health clinic. Interview clients about their means of transportation to reach health and social service agencies. Note the difficulties and identify resources that would be needed to improve access to these agencies.

INTERVIEWING AND RECORDING ASSESSMENT FINDINGS

Complete the following Community Assessment Checklist for a selected community. Choose a small community or a section of a larger community, for example an institution such as a university, a suburb, or an inner-city residential section. Analyze the data as indicated.

COMMUNITY ASSESSMENT CHECKLIST

Question	Normal findings	Abnormal findings	Additional data needed
Community of People			
1. Assess history.			
2. Assess age/gender.			
3. Assess racial/ethnic groups.			
4. Assess vital statistics (birth and death records).			
5. Assess household size/marital status/mobility.			
6. Assess values/religious beliefs.			

COMMUNITY ASSESSMENT CHECKLIST

Question	Normal findings	Abnormal findings	Additional data needed

Physical Environment

1. Assess geographic boundaries.

2. Assess neighborhoods.

3. Assess housing.

4. Assess climate and terrain.

Health and Social Services

1. Assess hospitals/clinics/emergency care/private practitioners.

2. Assess public health and home services.

3. Assess social service agencies.

4. Assess long-term care.

5. Assess economics.

6. Assess safety.

7. Assess transportation.

8. Assess education.

9. Assess government and politics.

10. Assess communication.

11. Assess recreation.

Analysis of Data

1. Formulate nursing diagnoses (wellness, risk, and actual).

2. Formulate collaborative problems.

3. Make necessary referrals.

CRITICAL THINKING AND CASE STUDIES

1. On the basis of the following assessment information, work through the steps of analyzing the data. Identify abnormal data and strengths in **subjective and objective findings**, assemble **cue clusters**, **draw inferences**, make possible **nursing diagnoses**, identify **defining characteristics**, **confirm or rule out** the nursing diagnosis, and **document** your conclusions.

   Use the blank diagnostic analysis charts provided at the end of this book to guide your thinking. You may want to write on the chart or use separate paper. Propose nursing diagnoses that are specific to the client in the case study. Identify collaborative problems, if any, for this client. Finally, identify data, if any, that point toward a medical problem requiring a referral.

History

The area known as Evansboro was first settled by French explorers and established as a military outpost. Soon afterward, the area was settled by other French immigrants because of its rich farmland. It was a busy trading post in the 1800s because of its location on the St. Croix River.

Demographics

The total population of Evansboro, as of the 2000 census, was 9,156. Of the total residents, the female-to-male ratio is 1.1:1. There are 1,767 persons who are 65 years of age or older, and 2,287 who are 18 years or younger. Racial distribution data reveal that 64.2% of the residents are African American, 34.5% are Caucasian, 0.8% are Native American, and 0.5% belong to other racial groups. Most of Evansboro's residents are married (71.6%), 23.1% are single, and the remainder are either separated, divorced, or widowed. The leading causes of death are cardiovascular disease and lung cancer. Several religious denominations are represented in Evansboro; those with the greatest percentage of members include Southern Baptist, African Methodist Episcopal, and United Methodist.

Physical

Evansboro is bordered on the west by the St. Croix River and is otherwise surrounded by farmland. It lies within the flood plain of the river and as a result is periodically threatened by flooding. The last time that homes were affected by flood waters was 3 years ago. Evansboro is located in Washington County. State Highway 25 borders the eastern limits of the town and intersects with U.S. Highway 62 along the northern border of Evansboro. The average temperature during the month of January is 60.3 degrees F; during the month of July it is 95.1 degrees F.

Health and Social Services

Evansboro has a small 50-bed general hospital with a 5-bed special care unit, an emergency room, and limited surgical services. No obstetric services are available. The hospital also provides hospice and home health services. Additional home health services are provided to the area through Housecalls, Inc. Twelve physicians provide services in Evansboro; seven are family practice specialists and the others include an internist, two pediatricians, and two general surgeons. There also are four dentists and three optometrists. The main office of the Washington County Health Department is in Evansboro and offers several services, including Women, Infants, and Children (WIC), immunizations, surveillance for sexually transmitted diseases (STDs), screening for chronic diseases, and a smoking cessation program. The health department does not provide family planning services and does not currently employ an environmental sanitarian. There is a small community counseling center that employs three full-time counselors, one full-time psychologist, and one part-time psychiatrist. Evansboro is the county seat and offers limited social welfare programs through government agencies such as Family and Children's Services. There are two long-term care facilities (with 100 beds and 65 beds), and both provide skilled nursing care. The county provides ambulance/EMT service but does not have a 911 system in place. The community has a Meals on Wheels program for the homebound. Civic and fraternal organizations, such as the Lions Club and the Business and Professional Women's Club, provide many services as well.

Economics

The median household income for Evansboro is $28,586; the median individual income is $15,356. Of the total population of Evansboro, 5.6% fall below the federal poverty guidelines. The major occupations in Evansboro are manufacturing, farming, and business, including agribusiness. The major crops include peanuts and tobacco. The manufacturers include Johnson's Peanut Processing Plant, Jordan Tobacco, Inc., and Pinewood Paper Mill. None of these companies employs a health nurse. The unemployment rate is 6.9%, which is near the state average.

Safety and Transportation

Evansboro employs seven full-time and four part-time policemen. The most frequently reported crimes are domestic assault, traffic violations, and vandalism. The crime rate is slightly lower than that for the state. The police department provides the D.A.R.E. program to the local middle school. The local fire department includes six full-time and six part-time employees and has recently purchased a new fire truck. There are also several volunteers trained by the fire department who offer their services when needed. The primary means of transportation is the private automobile. There is a taxi service in Evansboro, and the local senior citizen's center provides transportation to seniors within the city. There is a small county airport about 15 miles away, which provides commuter service to larger airports in the region.

Education

There are three elementary schools (grades K through 3), one middle school (grades 4 through 6), one junior high school (grades 7 and 8), and one senior high school (grades 9 through 12). Together the schools have an enrollment of approximately 1,900 students. One school nurse provides services for the three elementary schools, one nurse provides services between the middle school and the junior high school, and one school nurse is employed at the high school. The elementary and middle schools have an after-school program, and all schools have a school lunch program. The schools require physical education for all grades. The junior high offers programs in softball, baseball, basketball, and track. The high school also offers these same athletic programs as well as golf, wrestling, football, and volleyball. There is a variety of other extracurricular school-sponsored activities as well. The nurses employed at the high school and the junior high expressed some concern about what they believe is a growing problem with illicit drug and alcohol use among students. The high school offers GED classes, and the district's junior college, which is 30 miles away, offers some night classes in Evansboro. There is a community library, which is open 6 days a week. School officials and others in Evansboro are concerned about the condition of the junior high, which was built 70 years ago; the building is in need of many repairs and cannot adequately accommodate the number of students enrolled. The school board is considering a school bond referendum but is not optimistic because of the reluctance of voters to pass any tax increase.

Recreation

Evansboro has a city park with ball fields, tennis courts, soccer fields, picnic facilities, hiking trails, and a municipal pool. The park district provides several programs, including Red Cross swimming instruction, water aerobics for seniors, a swim team, Little League baseball and softball, soccer teams, and a tag football program for children aged 8 to 14. Evansboro has a movie theater, a bowling alley, a senior citizen's center, and several Boy Scout and Girl Scout troops. There are several other activities, such as the county fair and "Christmas in the Park," when businesses in town provide a light display in the city park. Other special-interest groups include a fishing club, a 4-H club, and a club for those interested in collecting. Church groups also offer a variety of recreational opportunities.

Politics and Government

Evansboro has an aldermanic type of local government. The city council is composed of eight elected members, two from each ward. The chair of the council is the mayor, who is also elected. There is a city attorney, a city treasurer, and a city clerk. The mayor is quite positive about the ability of the city council members to work together as well as about the response of the community to the city government. Both major political parties are represented in the city.

Communication

Evansboro has one local AM radio station, which primarily broadcasts local news and country music, and various other AM and FM stations broadcast in the area. There is a weekly newspaper, the *Evansboro Chronicle*. The city has cable television access, and Internet services are provided through Apex Internet, Inc. Evansboro has a post office and telephone services.

■ Chapter Post-test

MULTIPLE CHOICE QUESTIONS

Choose the one best answer for each of the following multiple-choice questions.

_____ 1. From a sociologic perspective, a community is defined as a group, population, or cluster of people with

A. common geographic boundaries.

B. a time-space relationship.

C. similar religious practices.

D. at least one common characteristic.

_____ 2. The definition of a community as defined by the World Health Organization includes

A. a community functioning within a particular social structure.

B. an open social system that is characterized by people in a place.

C. a cluster of people with similar political preferences.

D. a group of people with at least one common characteristic.

_____ 3. One example of a boundary for a geopolitical community is a

A. religious organization.

B. special-interest group.

C. subway system.

D. river.

_____ 4. The "Community as Partner" model is based on the work by the nursing theorist

A. Madeline Leininger.

B. Sister Callista Roy.

C. Imogene King.

D. Betty Neuman.

_____ 5. The nurse is assessing demographic information about a particular community. To assess the risk factors for health-related problems, the nurse should assess the community members'

A. ethnicity.

B. age.

C. housing density.

D. growth within the population.

_____ 6. A nurse is assessing a community of Native Americans. One important piece of health-related information that the nurse should obtain is the incidence of

A. tuberculosis.

B. congenital abnormalities.

C. pregnancy-induced hypertension.

D. diabetes mellitus.

_____ 7. In 1991, the number one cause of infant mortality in the United States was

A. sudden infant death syndrome.

B. low birth weight/prematurity.

C. respiratory distress syndrome.

D. congenital anomalies.

_____ 8. In 1993, the number one cause of childhood mortality in the United States for children between the ages of 1 and 4 years was

A. unintentional injuries.

B. malignant neoplasms.

C. homicide.

D. birth defects.

_____ 9. Occupational-related deaths and injuries in the United States are usually due to

  A. musculoskeletal injuries.

  B. burns.

  C. chemical injuries.

  D. poisonings.

_____ 10. In the assessment of a community, it is important for the nurse to assess the educational institutions. One indicator that there are problems in the high school system is the

  A. low absenteeism of the teachers.

  B. number of GED programs available.

  C. special education programs available.

  D. low graduation rate.

_____ 11. After assessing a local community, the nurse determines that there is a lack of community areas for exercise and socialization, particularly for the elderly members of the population. A priority nursing diagnosis for this community

  A. potential for enhanced community coping.

  B. ineffective community coping related to lack of funding.

  C. ineffective management of therapeutic regimen related to elderly population.

  D. risk for social isolation related to a lack of recreational activities and facilities.

▪ Self-Reflection and Evaluation of Learner Objectives

After you have read Chapter 28 and completed the above quizzes and activities, please identify to what degree you have met each of the following chapter learning objectives. For those objectives that you have met partially or not at all, you will want to review chapter content for that learning objective.

Objective	Very much	Somewhat	Not at all
1. Discuss how the history of a community may impact its current health status.			
2. Describe the types of demographic information necessary to complete a community assessment and the sources of this information.			
3. Discuss ways in which cultural and religious values affect health behaviors and attitudes.			
4. Describe factors that make up the physical environment of the community.			
5. Describe types of primary care facilities and providers that should be available in a community.			

Objective	Very much	Somewhat	Not at all
6. Discuss the types of programs/services that public health/home agencies can provide.			
7. Describe the types of agencies needed to provide necessary services within a community.			
8. Describe types of long-term care options that may be available in a community.			
9. Discuss how economic factors can affect health of a community.			
10. Describe services and programs essential to provide for the safety needs of a community (pp. 783-786).			
11. Discuss forms of transportation that may be available in a community and how lack of adequate transportation may impact health.			
12. Assess education-related factors in a community, and discuss the relationship between education and health.			
13. Describe the relationship of government officials and leaders to the overall welfare of the community.			
14. Identify formal and informal means of communication that may exist within a community.			
15. Describe ways in which recreation affects the health of individuals in a community			

For additional information on this book, be sure to visit *http://connection.lww.com.*

Answer Key

Chapter 1. The Nurse's Role in Health Assessment

CHAPTER PRETEST
Matching
1. F
2. I
3. A
4. B
5. E
6. G
7. C
8. J
9. H
10. D

CHAPTER POST-TEST
Multiple Choice
1. physiologic status.
2. D. formulation of nursing diagnoses.
3. A. continuous.
4. D. comprehensive.
5. D. includes a brief reassessment of the client's normal body system.
6. C. review the client's health care record.
7. C. avoid premature judgments about the client.
8. A. arrive at conclusions about the client's health.
9. D. check for the presence of defining characteristics.
10. B. rapid advances in biomedical knowledge and technology.

Chapter 2. Assessment Frameworks

CHAPTER PRETEST
Matching
1. D
2. F
3. A
4. H
5. I
6. C
7. E
8. G
9. B

CHAPTER POST-TEST
Multiple Choice
1. C. identify patterns of functioning that conform to or deviate from norms.
2. A. a set of abstract, interrelated statements.

3. D. Betty Newman.
4. A. Sister Callista Roy.
5. B. Imogene King.
6. D. Martha Rogers.
7. A. self-care agent who performs or practices activities to maintain life, health, and well-being.
8. D. "What is your typical daily food intake?"
9. A. values.
10. D. socialization.

Chapter 3. The Client in Context: Culture, Family, and Community

CHAPTER PRETEST
Multiple Choice
1. B. setting, environment.
2. D. All nursing conceptual frameworks consider the interacting systems of client and context.

True/False
1. T
2. T
3. T
4. a. T
   b. T
   c. T
   d. T
   e. T
   f. T
   g. F
   h. F
   i. T
5. T
6. T
7. F
8. T

CHAPTER POST-TEST
Multiple Choice
1. A. the belief that one's cultural values are superior to all others.
2. Do's and don'ts
   a. do
   b. don't
   c. don't
   d. do
   e. do
   f. do
   g. do

3. D. Community is the context in which health care professionals care for clients.

4. A. There is an interaction of culture, family, and environmental systems with the client's emotional and physical systems affecting the client's health status.

Matching

1. C
2. A
3. B
4. E
5. F
6. G
7. D

Chapter 4. Collecting Subjective Data

CHAPTER PRETEST
Multiple Choice

1. A. perception of pain.

2. D. using closed-ended questions.

3. A. acknowledge the client's cultural differences.

4. C. knowledge of his or her own thoughts and feelings about these issues.

5. A. use very basic lay terminology.

6. D. encourage the client to quit smoking.

7. A. avoids excessive eye contact with the client.

8. B. provide the client with information as questions arise.

9. A. maintain eye contact while asking the questions from the form.

10. A. assess the client's hearing acuity.

CHAPTER POST-TEST
Multiple Choice

1. B. rephrasing the client's statements.

2. C. working.

3. D. explain the role and purpose of the nurse.

4. A. allow the client to ventilate his feelings.

5. D. expressing interest in a neutral manner.

6. B. provide structure and set limits with the client.

7. D. identify risk factors to the client and his or her significant others.

8. B. review the food pyramid with the client.

9. D. "How do you manage your stress?"

Matching

1. G
2. D
3. B

4. H
5. F
6. A
7. C
8. E

Chapter 5. Collecting Objective Data

CHAPTER PRETEST
Matching

1. B
2. C
3. D
4. F
5. H
6. K
7. G
8. I
9. A
10. J
11. E

CHAPTER POST-TEST
Multiple Choice

1. A. wash both hands with soap and water.

2. B. explain each procedure being performed and the reason for the procedure.

3. D. use minimal position changes during the examination.

4. D. inspection.

5. C. dorsal surface of the hand.

6. C. deep palpation.

7. D. percussion.

8. D. blunt percussion.

9. D. blunt percussion.

10. C. indirect percussion.

11. A. hyperresonance.

12. B. bone.

13. B. 1 1/2-inch diaphragm.

Chapter 6. Validating and Documenting Data

CHAPTER PRETEST
Multiple Choice

1. D. draw a line through the error, writing "error" and initialing.

2. B. avoid slang terms or labels unless they are direct quotes.

3. A. "Bilateral lung sounds clear."

4. D. vital signs.

5. D. pain relief measures.

6. C. requires a lot of time to complete.

7. A. prevents missed questions during data collection.

8. B. may be easily used by different levels of caregivers, which enhances communication.

9. A. establishes comparability of nursing data across clinical populations.

10. D. focused.

11. A. validate all data before documentation of the data.

Matching

1. S
2. O
3. S
4. O
5. O
6. S
7. O
8. O
9. S
10. O

Chapter 7. Using Diagnostic Reasoning Skills to Analyze Data

CHAPTER PRETEST
Matching

1. F
2. E
3. A
4. B
5. H
6. I
7. C
8. D
9. G

CHAPTER POST-TEST
Multiple Choice

1. D. validate information and judgments.

2. D. perform the steps of the assessment process accurately.

3. A. fatigue related to excessive noise levels AMB client's statements of chronic fatigue.

4. D. quickly make a diagnosis without hypothesizing several diagnoses.

Chapter 8. General Survey and Nutritional Assessment

CHAPTER PRETEST
Multiple Choice

1. C. poor.

2. A. decreased body metabolism.

Matching

1. C
2. F
3. E
4. G
5. B
6. H
7. D
8. A

CHAPTER POST-TEST
Multiple Choice

1. C. vital signs.

2. A. normal changes that occur with the aging process.

3. B. observe for equal bilateral chest expansion of 1 to 2 inches.

4. A. shorter inspiratory phase.

5. C. "Are you having pain from your surgery?"

6. B. 30 to 50 mm Hg.

7. D. imbalanced nutrition: more than body requirements.

8. A. heart attack.

9. D. repeat the procedure three times and average the measurements.

Chapter 9. Skin, Hair, and Nail Assessment

CHAPTER PRETEST
Multiple Choice

1. D. subcutaneous tissue.

2. D. D.

3. A. innermost layer of the epidermis.

4. B. volume of blood circulating in the dermis.

5. D. dermis.

6. A. areola of the breast.

7. A. vellus.

8. B. filter for dust.

9. C. keratinized epidermal cells.

CHAPTER POST-TEST
Multiple Choice

1. D. domestic abuse.

2. A. symptoms of stress.

3. D. squamous cell carcinomas are most common on body sites with heavy sun exposure.

4. A. overall amount of sun exposure.

5. C. chronic discoid lupus erythematosus.

6. A. hypothyroidism.

7. D. malignant melanoma.

8. D. fluid intake.

9. B. oral mucosa.

10. B. ashen.

11. A. a great degree of cyanosis.

12. D. sclera.

13. B. due to aging of the skin in older adults.

14. A. blue.

15. B. Stage II.

16. D. use two fingers to pinch the skin under the clavicle.

17. C. a recent illness.

18. A. hypoxia.

19. A. macules.

20. A. plaque.

21. C. vesicles.

22. D. fissures.

23. D. keloid.

24. D. risk for ineffective health maintenance related to deficient knowledge of effects of sunlight on skin lesions.

Crossword Puzzle

Crossword puzzle answers appear on page 289.

Chapter 10. Head and Neck Assessment

CHAPTER PRETEST
Matching

1. D
2. H
3. A
4. I
5. B
6. F
7. C
8. E
9. J
10. G

CHAPTER POST-TEST
Multiple Choice

1. A. reduction of the blood supply to the brain.

2. B. meningeal irritation.

3. D. trigeminal neuralgia.

4. A. migraine headache.

5. A. cluster headaches.

6. D. tension headaches.

7. D. tumor-related headache.

8. B. ask the client if touching the head is permissible.

9. B. acromegaly.

10. C. Paget's disease.

11. D. parotid gland enlargement.

12. B. swallow a small sip of water.

13. C. refer the client to a physician for further evaluation.

14. B. approach the client posteriorly.

15. D. sit in an upright position.

16. C. health-seeking behaviors related to verbalization of wanting to stay healthy.

Chapter 11. Eye Assessment

CHAPTER PRETEST
Multiple Choice

1. C. protector.

2. A. meibomian glands.

3. D. bulbar portion.

4. D. rectus muscles.

5. A. choroid layer.

6. C. retina.

7. A. an oily substance to lubricate the eyes.

8. D. cleanse the cornea and the lens.

9. A. optic chiasma.

10. B. accommodation.

CHAPTER POST-TEST
Multiple Choice

1. D. corneal reflexes.

2. D. head trauma.

3. C. check the client's blood pressure.

4. A. tell the client that these often occur with aging.

5. A. glaucoma.

6. B. refer the client to an ophthalmologist.

7. D. vitamin A deficiency.

8. B. increased intracranial pressure.

9. D. allergies.

10. D. a foreign body in the eye.

11. D. lacrimal obstruction.

12. B. 2 years.

13. D. corneal damage.

14. B. ultraviolet light exposure.

15. A. position the client 20 feet away from the chart.

16. D. refer the client to an optometrist.

17. D. document the findings in the client's records.
18. B. decreased accommodation.
19. A. esotropia.
20. C. requires the covering of each eye separately.

Chapter 12. Ear Assessment

CHAPTER PRETEST
Multiple Choice

1. C. external ear.
2. D. stapes.
3. A. vestibule.
4. A. fluid.
5. B. conductive hearing.
6. D. perceptive hearing.

CHAPTER POST-TEST
Multiple Choice

1. C. taking antibiotics.
2. C. "It is difficult to prevent hearing loss or worsening of hearing."
3. D. observe the client's response to the explanations.
4. D. firmly pull the auricle out, up, and back.
5. D. refer the client to a physician.
6. A. infection.
7. D. strike a tuning fork and place it on the center of the client's head or forehead.
8. C. conductive hearing loss.

Matching

1. G
2. I
3. A
4. C
5. E
6. D
7. H
8. B
9. F

Chapter 13. Mouth, Nose, Throat, and Sinus Assessment

CHAPTER PRETEST
Multiple Choice

1. D. soft palate.
2. A. uvula.
3. B. frenulum.
4. C. Wharton's ducts.
5. D. warm the inspired air.

CHAPTER POST-TEST
Multiple Choice

1. maxillary sinuses.
2. D. aphthous stomatitis.
3. A. refer the client for further evaluation.
4. D. refer the client for further evaluation.
5. A. aspiration.
6. D. stress and anxiety.
7. A. Diets low in fruits and vegetables are a possible risk factor for oral cancer.
8. D. don clean gloves for the procedure.
9. D. riboflavin.
10. A. *Candida albicans* infection.
11. B. area underneath the tongue.
12. A. depress the tongue blade slightly off center.
13. C. touching each other.
14. A. position the handle of the otoscope to one side.
15. D. an upper respiratory infection.

Matching

1. E
2. H
3. M
4. J
5. P
6. C
7. K
8. N
9. B
10. G
11. I
12. A
13. F
14. L
15. D
16. O

Chapter 14. Thoracic and Lung Assessment

CHAPTER PRETEST
Multiple Choice

1. D. manubrium.
2. A. angle.
3. C. Seventh.
4. B. area slightly above the clavicle.
5. A. parietal pleura.
6. D. cilia.
7. D. hypercapnia.

CHAPTER POST-TEST
Multiple Choice

1. D. infection.
2. D. tuberculosis.
3. D. Studies have indicated that there is a genetic component in the development of lung cancer.
4. D. chronic obstructive pulmonary disease.
5. D. asking the client to exhale forcefully and hold his breath.
6. C. ask the client to breathe deeply through her mouth.
7. A. repeat the phrase "ninety-nine."
8. B. pectus excavatum.
9. A. chronic bronchitis.
10. A. pneumonia.
11. D. bronchitis.
12. A. diabetic ketoacidosis.

Matching

1. D
2. G
3. J
4. H
5. B
6. I
7. C
8. F
9. A
10. E

Chapter 15. Breast and Lymphatic Assessment

CHAPTER PRETEST
Multiple Choice

1. A. progesterone.
2. D. areolas.
3. B. glandular.
4. D. Cooper's ligaments.
5. D. fatty tissue.
6. A. lateral lymph nodes.

CHAPTER POST-TEST
Multiple Choice

1. C upper outer quadrant.
2. C fibrocystic breast disease.
3. A having a baby before the age of 20 years.
4. C physical stress.
5. D breast cancer patients of the same race.
6. D contraceptives.

7. B depression.
8. D grapefruit juice.
9. D right after menstruation.
10. A blocked lymphatic drainage.
11. C refer the client for a cytology examination
12. B tumor.
13. C an infectious process.
14. D disturbed body image related to mastectomy.

Matching

1. I
2. F
3. L
4. H
5. D
6. M
7. K
8. B
9. E
10. N
11. A
12. J
13. G
14. C

Chapter 16. Heart and Neck Vessel Assessment

CHAPTER PRETEST
Multiple Choice

1. A. precordium.
2. A. between the left atrium and the left ventricle.
3. A. at the exit of each ventricle at the beginning of the great vessels.
4. A. posterior wall of the right atrium.
5. A. conduction of the impulse throughout the atria.

CHAPTER POST-TEST
Multiple Choice

1. C. apex of the heart.
2. D. can be heard during diastole.
3. B. angina.
4. A. high serum level of low-density lipoproteins.
5. D. Estrogen replacement therapy in postmenopausal women decreases the risk of heart attack.
6. A. apical pulse.
7. A. ask the client to hold her breath.
8. C. associated with occlusive arterial disease.
9. D. increased central venous pressure.
10. A. cardiac murmur.

11. B. third to fifth intercostal space at the left sternal border.

12. D. refer the client to a physician.

13. D. recognize that this finding is normal in adolescents.

14. C. mitral valve stenosis.

15. A. obstructive lung disease.

16. D. heart rate speeds up and slows down during a cycle.

17. A. low-frequency sound best heard with the bell of the stethoscope.

Crossword Puzzle

Crossword puzzle answers appear on page 289.

Chapter 17. Peripheral Vascular Assessment

CHAPTER PRETEST
Multiple Choice

1. D. brachial artery.
2. A. knee.
3. D. ankle.
4. C. 70%.

CHAPTER POST-TEST
Multiple Choice

1. D. arterial insufficiency.
2. A. venous insufficiency.
3. B. intermittent claudication.
4. D. getting regular exercise.
5. A. apply K-Y jelly to the client's skin.
6. A. lymphedema.
7. C. brachial pulse.
8. C. flex his elbow about 90 degrees.
9. D. venous insufficiency.
10. D. malignancy.
11. D. flex the client's knee, then dorsiflex the foot.
12. C. competence of saphenous vein valves.

Matching

1. I
2. D
3. K
4. M
5. G
6. L
7. B
8. J

9. F
10. C
11. E
12. A
13. H

Chapter 18. Abdominal Assessment

CHAPTER PRETEST
Multiple Choice

1. C. abdominal oblique.
2. B. left lower quadrant.
3. D. deep in the upper abdomen and is not normally palpable.
4. A. store and excrete bile.
5. A. right lower quadrant.

CHAPTER POST-TEST
Multiple Choice

1. A. right upper quadrant.
2. D. right lower quadrant.
3. B. left upper quadrant.
4. D. costovertebral angle.
5. A. stomach ulcers.
6. C. appetite changes.
7. A. "I can decrease the constipation if I eat foods high in fiber and drink water."
8. C. disturbed body image related to temporary colostomy.
9. D. inspect the abdominal area.
10. A. ask the client to empty his bladder.
11. D. internal bleeding.
12. D. masses.
13. A. umbilical hernia.
14. D. peritoneal irritation.
15. B. paralytic ileus.
16. A. intestinal obstruction.
17. C. use the diaphragm of the stethoscope.
18. B. place the right hand below the left costal margin.
19. D. palpate deeply while quickly releasing pressure.
20. C. raise the client's right leg from the hip.

Chapter 19. Male Genitalia Assessment

CHAPTER PRETEST
Multiple Choice

1. A. glans.
2. D. foreskin.
3. B. suspended by the spermatic cord.
4. A. just above and parallel to the inguinal ligament.

CHAPTER POST-TEST
Multiple Choice

1. D. prostate enlargement.
2. C. 3 years.
3. A. transient periods of erectile dysfunction are common.
4. C. inguinal hernia.
5. D. has anal intercourse with other males.
6. D. continue the examination in an unhurried manner.
7. A. ask the client to empty his bladder.
8. B. herpes infection.
9. B. syphilis
10. A. urethritis.
11. C. cryptorchidism.
12. C. epididymitis.
13. D. varicocele.
14. D. bowel sounds at the bulge.
15. A. refer the client to an emergency room.

Matching

1. C
2. E
3. G
4. F
5. A
6. H
7. B
8. D

Chapter 20. Female Genitalia Assessment

CHAPTER PRETEST
Multiple Choice

1. C. sweat glands.
2. D. glans.
3. A. vestibule.
4. A. pink squamous epithelium and connective tissue.
5. D. estrogen.

CHAPTER POST-TEST
Multiple Choice

1. B. "Do you experience mood swings or bloating?"
2. A. hot flashes.
3. D. infection.
4. B. sexually transmitted disease.
5. A. decreased urethral elasticity.
6. A. refrain from douching 48 hours before the examination.
7. C. warm tap water.
8. A. bear down.
9. D. cystocele.
10. A. stress incontinence.
11. A. infection.
12. A. herpes simplex virus infection.
13. D. genital warts.
14. A. *Trichomonas vaginalis* infection.
15. D. ectopic pregnancy.

Matching

1. G
2. E
3. K
4. F
5. C
6. H
7. L
8. B
9. J
10. D
11. A
12. I

Chapter 21. Anus, Rectum, and Prostate Assessment

CHAPTER PRETEST
Multiple Choice

1. A. composed of smooth muscle.
2. D. intersphincteric groove.
3. D. hemorrhoids.
4. A. median sulcus.
5. B. secrete a milky substance that neutralizes female acidic secretions.
6. C. empty into the urethra.

CHAPTER POST-TEST
Multiple Choice

1. A. gastrointestinal infection.
2. D. gastrointestinal bleeding.

3. A. biliary disease.

4. A. year.

5. C. Diets high in fat and low in fiber are associated with colorectal cancer.

6. D. advanced age.

7. A. African-American

8. B. left lateral position.

9. D. bear down.

10. C. a fungal infection.

11. C. pilonidal cysts.

12. A. polyps.

13. D. peritoneal metastasis.

14. A. prostate cancer.

Matching

1. F
2. D
3. L
4. J
5. H
6. B
7. I
8. E
9. K
10. C
11. A
12. G

Chapter 22. Musculoskeletal Assessment

CHAPTER PRETEST
Multiple Choice

1. C. produce blood cells.

2. A. fat.

3. D. periosteum.

4. A. tendons.

5. D. fibrous.

6. B. ligaments.

7. D. abduction.

8. A. supination.

9. B. shoulder joint.

10. D. hip joint.

CHAPTER POST-TEST
Multiple Choice Questions

1. A. arthritis.

2. C. osteomyelitis.

3. A. osteoporosis.

4. C. Moderate strenuous exercise tends to increase bone density.

5. D. vitamin C.

6. A. gouty arthritis.

7. D. vitamin D.

8. D. "You'll continue with range of motion even if I have discomfort."

9. C. average weakness.

10. B. TMJ dysfunction.

11. A. herniated disc.

12. D. scoliosis.

13. D. lie flat and raise his leg to the point of pain.

14. A. herniated intervertebral disc.

15. A. rotator cuff tear.

16. C. calcified tendinitis.

17. D. XI.

18. A. arthritis.

19. D. inability to extend the ring and little finger.

20. A. osteoarthritis.

21. D. place the backs of both hands against each other.

22. B. carpal tunnel syndrome.

23. D. synovitis.

24. A. place the left thumb and index finger on either side of the patella.

25. C. osteoarthritis.

26. D. flex the knee and hip while in a supine position.

27. A. hallux valgus.

28. D. flat feet.

29. D. gouty arthritis.

30. A. hammer toes.

31. C. plantar warts.

Crossword Puzzle

Crossword puzzle answers appear on page 289.

Chapter 23. Neurologic Assessment

CHAPTER PRETEST
Multiple Choice

1. D. removes wastes.

2. A. corpus callosum.

3. A. gray matter.

4. D. thalamus and hypothalamus.

5. A. sleep cycles.

Matching

1. B.
2. E.
3. H.
4. L.
5. G.
6. K.
7. C.
8. A.
9. J.
10. D.
11. I .
12. F.

CHAPTER POST-TEST
Multiple Choice

1. spinothalamic tract.
2 . D. glossopharyngeal.
3. B. cerebral vascular accident.
4. B. Smoking and high cholesterol levels are risk factors for CVA.
5. A. sensation in the extremities.
6. A. clench his jaw.
7. D. some impairment.
8. A. depression.
9. D. cerebral cortex disorder.
10. D. "Can you repeat *brown, chair, textbook, tomato?*"
11. A. oculomotor nerve paralysis.
12. A. ask the client to purse the lips.
13. D. corticospinal tract.
14. C. stand erect with arms at the sides and feet together.
15. B. toes up or down.
16. D. document the finding in the client's record.
17. C. drug intoxication.

Chapter 24. Assessment of Infants, Children, and Adolescents

CHAPTER PRETEST
Multiple Choice

1. D. smooth-textured skin.
2. D. 12 and 18 months.
3. A. A child's head reaches 90% of its full growth by 6 years of age.
4. A. is an obligatory nose breather.
5. C. fourth intercostal space.

Matching

1. B
2. D
3. B
4. E
5. E
6. A
7. D
8. A
9. A
10. D
11. B
12. B
13. C
14. E
15. E
16. A
17. C
18. D
19. D
20. A

CHAPTER POST-TEST
Multiple Choice

1. B. three.
2. B. 12 and 18 months.
3. C. 14 years.
4. D. talk to the child in simple terms at the child's eye level.
5. A. play.
6. A. tell the child it is okay to cry in the clinic.
7. D. allow the child to engage in the discussions.
8. A. give the client control whenever possible.
9. C. oral polio vaccine, HiB, and DPT.
10. C. 24 pounds.
11. B. 6 years.
12. D. 30 months after the onset of puberty.
13. A. hop on one foot.
14. D. make simple classifications.
15. A. she can begin bowel training as soon as the child appears ready.
16. B. 4 to 6 months old.
17. A. cystic fibrosis.
18. A. document the finding in the client's record.
19. D. storkbite.
20. D. iron.
21. A. Epstein's pearls.
22. A. measles.
23. B. shine a light directly into the pupils.
24. A. down and back.

Chapter 25. Assessment of the Childbearing Woman

CHAPTER PRETEST
Multiple Choice

1. D. fade to a white or silvery color.
2. A. linea nigra.
3. D. progesterone.
4. C. is normal for some women in the second and third trimesters.
5. A. an increase in maternal blood volume by 40 to 50%.
6. D. diastasis recti abdominis.
7. A. "As a result of pregnancy, diarrhea may occur more often."
8. C. nutritional status.
9. A. estrogen.
10. C. at the level of the umbilicus.

LEARNER ACTIVITIES
Crossword Puzzle

Crossword puzzle answers appear on page 289.

CHAPTER POST-TEST
Multiple Choice

1. D. supine
2. C. 25 to 35 pounds.
3. A. hyperemesis gravidarum.
4. A. incompetent cervix.
5. D. Tay-Sachs disease.
6. D. abruptio placenta.
7. D. Rh status.
8. D. blood pressure.
9. A. upper quadrant of the maternal abdomen.
10. A. 10 weeks.
11. D. poor placental perfusion.
12. B. breech
13. A. gonorrhea.
14. C. pregnancy-induced hypertension.
15. A. instruct the client that a vaginal delivery is likely.

Chapter 26. Assessment of the Frail Elderly Adult

CHAPTER PRETEST
Multiple Choice

1. C. acute or chronic illness places excessive demands on the body.
2. D. lentigo.

3. C. postural instability.
4. B. confusion.
5. D. 50%.
6. B. a decrease in reaction time.

Matching

1. B
2. C
3. A
4. D

CHAPTER POST-TEST
Multiple Choice

1. A. a nasogastric feeding tube.
2. D. fever.
3. D. urinary tract infection.
4. B. a Get Up and Go test.
5. C. diverticulitis.
6. C. with the feet farther apart and the knees slightly bent.
7. D. cognitive impairment or pseudodementia.
8. C. the degree to which dyspnea affects daily function.
9. C. a rapid decline in level of alertness.
10. B. tenting of skin when pinched.
11. C. hair loss on the skin.

Matching
PART 1

1. D
2. B
3. A
4. C

PART 2

5. E, F
6. G, I, J
7. G, J
8. H
9. G, I

Chapter 27. Assessment of the Family

CHAPTER PRETEST
Multiple Choice

1. D. have mutual decision making.
2. A. the gender of the members.
3. D. mother–son.
4. D. rigid.
5. C. is shared by both parents.

Matching
1. D
2. E
3. B
4. C
5. A

CHAPTER POST-TEST
Multiple Choice
1. D. square.
2. A. ethnicity.
3. D. instrumental.
4. D. determining the boundaries of the subsystems in the family structure.
5. A. rigid patterns of interactions.
6. B. general systems theory.
7. C. oldest son marries youngest daughter.
8. A. neighborhood's safety.
9. D. socialization.
10. D. risk for dysfunctional grieving related to loss of health status of youthful family member

Matching
1. C
2. E
3. A
4. D
5. B

Chapter 28. Assessment of the Community

CHAPTER PRETEST
Multiple Choice
1. C. motor vehicle accidents.
2. D. cancer.

3. A. heart disease.
4. C. tripled.
5. C. role overload.
6. D. lack of affordable housing.
7. D. obstetric care.
8. D. home health care agencies.
9. C. a lack of transportation.
10. D. poverty.

Crossword Puzzle
Crossword puzzle answers appear on page 289.

CHAPTER POST-TEST
Multiple Choice
1. D. at least one common characteristic.
2. A. a community functioning within a particular social structure.
3. D. river.
4. D. Betty Neuman.
5. B. age.
6. D. diabetes mellitus.
7. D. congenital anomalies.
8. A. unintentional injuries.
9. A. musculoskeletal injuries.
10. D. low graduation rate.
11. D. risk for social isolation related to a lack of recreational activities and facilities.

Crossword Puzzle Answer Key

CHAPTER 9

Across

1. papule
7. induration
10. fissure
11. macule
12. diffuse
14. contusion
17. annular
20. tumor
22. excoriation
24. vesicle
25. petechiae

Down

1. pustule
2. plaque
3. erosion
4. nevus
5. lichenification
6. bulla
8. nodule
9. keloid
13. confluent
15. crust
16. atrophy
18. scale
19. urticaria
21. ulcer
23. wheal

CHAPTER 16

Across

1. pulmonic
4. diaphragm
6. infarct
9. auscultation
10. pedis
11. thrill
13. PMI
14. mitral
15. radial
17. systole
23. aortic
24. heave
26. splitting
27. bradycardia

Down

2. murmur
3. tibial
5. peripheral
6. ischemia
7. pulse
8. bekk
12. diastole
16. apex
18. tricuspid
19. ERBS
20. bruit
21. angina
22. thrombus
24. Homan's
25. NSR

CHAPTER 22

Across

1. range of motion
5. adduction
6. external
8. bursitis
10. clonus
11. ankylosis
14. myalgia
15. cogwheel
17. dorsiflexion
18. lordosis

Down

2. abduction
3. crepitus
4. flexion
7. circumduction
8. bursa
9. fasciculation
12. extension
13. kyphosis
16. plantar

CHAPTER 25

Across

1. ectopic
4. linea nigra
6. palpation
7. epulis
8. relaxin
9. back
10. 30
12. breech
13. chloasma
17. lie
18. false

Down

2. pica
3. striae gravidarum
4. Leopold's maneuvers
5. anemia
11. three
14. obstetric
15. ambivalent
16. colostrum
16. gynecoid

CHAPTER 28

Across

2. team
6. snow
8. pantries
11. morbidity
13. sickle cell
18. river
19. Census
21. Labor
22. mayor
23. DARE
25. vital
28. GED
29. waste
30. YMCA
31. transit
32. lake

Down

1. rural
3. MADD
4. SSA
5. cancer
7. WIC
9. EPA
10. ambulance
12. RR
13. SIDS
14. Lyme
15. Army
16. board
17. lead
20. survey
22. Meals
24. park
25. VNA
26. lore
27. DOT

APPENDIX:
Diagnostic Reasoning Guides

1 Identify abnormal data and strengths (in both subjective and objective data).

SUBJECTIVE DATA

OBJECTIVE DATA

2 Cue Clusters

3 Possible Nursing Inferences

4 Presence of Diagnosis

5 Defining Characteristics

6 Confirm or Rule Out

7 Document Conclusions

NURSING DIAGNOSES

COLLABORATIVE PROBLEMS

MEDICAL PROBLEMS

1 Identify abnormal data and strengths (in both subjective and objective data).

SUBJECTIVE DATA

OBJECTIVE DATA

2 Cue Clusters

3 Possible Nursing Inferences

4 Presence of Diagnosis

5 Defining Characteristics

6 Confirm or Rule Out

7 Document Conclusions

NURSING DIAGNOSES

COLLABORATIVE PROBLEMS

MEDICAL PROBLEMS

1. Identify abnormal data and strengths (in both subjective and objective data).

SUBJECTIVE DATA

OBJECTIVE DATA

2. Cue Clusters

3. Possible Nursing Inferences

4. Presence of Diagnosis

5. Defining Characteristics

6. Confirm or Rule Out

7. Document Conclusions

NURSING DIAGNOSES

COLLABORATIVE PROBLEMS

MEDICAL PROBLEMS

1 Identify abnormal data and strengths (in both subjective and objective data).

SUBJECTIVE DATA   **OBJECTIVE DATA**

2 Cue Clusters

3 Possible Nursing Inferences

4 Presence of Diagnosis

5 Defining Characteristics

6 Confirm or Rule Out

7 Document Conclusions

NURSING DIAGNOSES

COLLABORATIVE PROBLEMS

MEDICAL PROBLEMS

① Identify abnormal data and strengths (in both subjective and objective data).

SUBJECTIVE DATA

OBJECTIVE DATA

② Cue Clusters

③ Possible Nursing Inferences

④ Presence of Diagnosis

⑤ Defining Characteristics

⑥ Confirm or Rule Out

⑦ Document Conclusions

NURSING DIAGNOSES

COLLABORATIVE PROBLEMS

MEDICAL PROBLEMS

1 Identify abnormal data and strengths (in both subjective and objective data).

SUBJECTIVE DATA **OBJECTIVE DATA**

2 Cue Clusters

3 Possible Nursing Inferences

4 Presence of Diagnosis

5 Defining Characteristics

6 Confirm or Rule Out

7 Document Conclusions

NURSING DIAGNOSES

COLLABORATIVE PROBLEMS

MEDICAL PROBLEMS

1 Identify abnormal data and strengths (in both subjective and objective data).

SUBJECTIVE DATA

OBJECTIVE DATA

2 Cue Clusters

3 Possible Nursing Inferences

4 Presence of Diagnosis

5 Defining Characteristics

6 Confirm or Rule Out

7 Document Conclusions

NURSING DIAGNOSES

COLLABORATIVE PROBLEMS

MEDICAL PROBLEMS

1 Identify abnormal data and strengths (in both subjective and objective data).

SUBJECTIVE DATA

OBJECTIVE DATA

2 Cue Clusters

3 Possible Nursing Inferences

4 Presence of Diagnosis

5 Defining Characteristics

6 Confirm or Rule Out

7 Document Conclusions

NURSING DIAGNOSES

COLLABORATIVE PROBLEMS

MEDICAL PROBLEMS

1 Identify abnormal data and strengths (in both subjective and objective data).

SUBJECTIVE DATA

OBJECTIVE DATA

2 Cue Clusters

3 Possible Nursing Inferences

4 Presence of Diagnosis

5 Defining Characteristics

6 Confirm or Rule Out

7 Document Conclusions

NURSING DIAGNOSES

COLLABORATIVE PROBLEMS

MEDICAL PROBLEMS

1　Identify abnormal data and strengths (in both subjective and objective data).

SUBJECTIVE DATA　　**OBJECTIVE DATA**

2　Cue Clusters

3　Possible Nursing Inferences

4　Presence of Diagnosis

5　Defining Characteristics

6　Confirm or Rule Out

7　Document Conclusions

NURSING DIAGNOSES

COLLABORATIVE PROBLEMS

MEDICAL PROBLEMS

1 Identify abnormal data and strengths (in both subjective and objective data).

SUBJECTIVE DATA

OBJECTIVE DATA

2 Cue Clusters

3 Possible Nursing Inferences

4 Presence of Diagnosis

5 Defining Characteristics

6 Confirm or Rule Out

7 Document Conclusions

NURSING DIAGNOSES

COLLABORATIVE PROBLEMS

MEDICAL PROBLEMS

1 Identify abnormal data and strengths (in both subjective and objective data).

SUBJECTIVE DATA   **OBJECTIVE DATA**

2 Cue Clusters

3 Possible Nursing Inferences

4 Presence of Diagnosis

5 Defining Characteristics

6 Confirm or Rule Out

7 Document Conclusions

NURSING DIAGNOSES

COLLABORATIVE PROBLEMS

MEDICAL PROBLEMS

1 Identify abnormal data and strengths (in both subjective and objective data).

SUBJECTIVE DATA

OBJECTIVE DATA

2 Cue Clusters

3 Possible Nursing Inferences

4 Presence of Diagnosis

5 Defining Characteristics

6 Confirm or Rule Out

7 Document Conclusions

NURSING DIAGNOSES

COLLABORATIVE PROBLEMS

MEDICAL PROBLEMS

1 Identify abnormal data and strengths (in both subjective and objective data).

SUBJECTIVE DATA   **OBJECTIVE DATA**

2 Cue Clusters

3 Possible Nursing Inferences

4 Presence of Diagnosis

5 Defining Characteristics

6 Confirm or Rule Out

7 Document Conclusions

NURSING DIAGNOSES

COLLABORATIVE PROBLEMS

MEDICAL PROBLEMS

1 Identify abnormal data and strengths (in both subjective and objective data).

SUBJECTIVE DATA

OBJECTIVE DATA

2 Cue Clusters

3 Possible Nursing Inferences

4 Presence of Diagnosis

5 Defining Characteristics

6 Confirm or Rule Out

7 Document Conclusions

NURSING DIAGNOSES

COLLABORATIVE PROBLEMS

MEDICAL PROBLEMS

1 Identify abnormal data and strengths (in both subjective and objective data).

SUBJECTIVE DATA   **OBJECTIVE DATA**

2 Cue Clusters

3 Possible Nursing Inferences

4 Presence of Diagnosis

5 Defining Characteristics

6 Confirm or Rule Out

7 Document Conclusions

NURSING DIAGNOSES

COLLABORATIVE PROBLEMS

MEDICAL PROBLEMS